CELIAC DISEASE. NEW CAUSES ARE DISCOVERED.

Cereals are not the only protagonists.

Dr. Andrea Helena Passera

Doctor of Medicine, graduated from the Faculty of Medicine of the National University of Córdoba (Universidad Nacional de Córdoba, UNC). After completing her medical residency in Pediatrics at *Hospital de Niños de la Santísima Trinidad*, she worked on a research project about Coeliac Disease at the Chair of Electron Microscopy at the UNC. Currently working as a medical specialist in Pediatrics at Sanatorio Allende, Córdoba City.

ISBN-13: 978-1517720964

ISBN-10: 1517720966

To God, the source of my strength; my children, Francisco and Facundo; my husband, Fernando; and my parents, who lovingly accompany me in my dreams and projects; and my brother, Ricardo, who taught me how to study.

CONTENTS

ACKNOWLEDGMENTS

Special thanks to Prof. Dr. Agustín Aoki, who was my thesis supervisor and passed me his knowledge to do my work, monitored me and guided me to draft the contents of my thesis; Dr. Claudia Palmieri, a great friend of mine who selflessly accompanied me whenever I needed her during laboratory experimentation and who guided me during research and writing. To Dr. Mario Passera, my father, for whom I have great admiration and who taught me about food allergy, an area in which I consider him a great pioneer.

I would also like to thank the members of the thesis committee: Prof. Dr. Elsa Margarita Orgnero, and Prof. Dr. Daniel Quiroga, Prof. Dr. Ruth Fernandez, for her supervision and all the members of the Center for Electron Microscopy who worekd together to make these projects a reality, including Prof. Dr. Patricia Pons, Prof. Dr. Alicia Torres, Dr. Cristina Maldonado, and the wonderful team of other doctors, biochemists, biologists and technicians who made this possible. Thank you. To Cecilia de la Vega, a great writer and friend, for her advice, and the family at Sanatorio Allende, founder of the institution where I work every day, for encouraging doctors to seek continuous improvement.

Translator: Natalia Medail (nlmedail@gmail.com). Special thanks to translator Lis Stampfer (lis_stampfer@yahoo.co.uk) for her amazing collaboration during the translation of this work into English.

Andrea Helena Passera

ABBREVIATIONS

AG gliadin antibodies, AE endomysium antibodies, CD Celiac Disease, °C degree Celsius, ELISA enzyme linked immunoassay, fig figure, g gram, h hour, HRLM High Resolution Light Microscopy, Ig immunoglobulin , ml milliliter, nm nanometer, µg microgram, µL microliter, µm micrometer.

Andrea Helena Passera

FOREWORD

Celiac disease involves a web of complexities that are made tangible in the first difficulty, diagnosis. I consulted Dr. Passera, today "Andrea", a dear friend, in such a state of bewilderment and anguish that I could only think of one thing: I felt that as a mother, I was doing everything wrong. For years, my husband and I visited doctor after doctor to try to determine what was wrong with our children's health. Three little boys, at the time, 6, 4 and 2 years old, with different symptoms but much in common: the kids were not growing well, they did not feel well. Our children were constantly sick and looked pale.

This is how we Andrea and I began a rigorous analysis protocol, tests and dietary restrictions that led to the general diagnosis of allergy to cow's milk protein for the three boys and celiac disease for two of them. "Genetic predisposition", "cross-intolerance" were the words that Dr. Passera used to explain the situation with the professionalism and humanity that define her. My three children stopped consuming dairy and beef and the two little ones began a gluten-free diet. The diagnosis of the boys resulted in another revelation: I was also celiac. Shortly after I had the tests done, I joined the boys with their gluten-free diet. There is so far no cure for CD. We know that. However, we do not consider ourselves "sick" because we never saw this that way. Our youngest children are "gluten-free" as they usually introduce themselves. Today, with this diet, the boys are healthy and full of color. Being able to understand what happened to them and adjust our life to their condition changed their lives and the life of our whole family.

The book that I have the honor of presenting today helps us better understand the implications of celiac disease. And the possibility of understanding allows us to act, change and improve. Cereals with glutamine are not the only ones to blame for celiac disease. Wheat, oats, barley and rye are just some of the factors, amongst others, that come together in the development of this disease. In her research, Dr. Passera clearly and forcefully sets out ample evidence that dairy products and some oils also crucially affect the onset and progression of celiac disease.

Understanding that celiac patients are affected not only by gluten intake allows us to see that the consequences of the so-called "cross-contamination" widely feared by the celiac community can have multiple causes. The fact that a celiac patient on an strict gluten-free diet continues to experience symptoms of the disease, or that their antibody tests continue to show positive results, may not be linked to the fact that they have eaten something "contaminated" or that a crumb of bread slipped on their plate; it can mean that it is very likely that they may suffer the consequences of eating other foods that contribute to the development of the disease.

The work of Dr. Passera breaks new ground in the study of the celiac disease. It broadens the range of factors that should be considered to improve the quality of life of celiac patients and sheds a light of hope in the treatment of the celiac disease. There is still much to discover and investigate about this disease. There are other variables in our diet, in addition to cereals, which we, celiac patients, can control to feel better and better. The roads are not closed, they are not final. And this can only be good.

María Cecilia De la Vega
English teacher and translator
Professor of the School of Languages
National University of Córdoba

PRESENTATION

I was at Lucia's birthday party when a classmate arrived with his mother. When the mother was leaving the girl, she said worried and briskly, "Please, do not let my daughter drink from another child's glass because she suffers from celiac disease". Those words echoed in my head during the day and in dreams at night, until once, Dr. Augustine Aoki, a valuable researcher of our university, motivated me to start my research which would eventually end up in my Doctoral Thesis. I have always worked as a pediatrician and while working in a lab scared me a bit, I began to feel more and more excited about it, which eventually resulted in the work that I share in this book. Obviously, I chose the subject of my thesis based on a question I always ask myself: Can a crumb change the status of a celiac patient or are there other elements of the diet that combine with gluten in the development of the disease?

The pathogenesis of celiac disease (CD) is and has been the target of numerous investigations; however, there are still many problems that remain unsolved. In the last decade new concepts related to the age of onset of symptoms, forms of presentation and the incidence of the disease were established. The cause of CD is usually attributed to the toxicity of prolamin of wheat. Today is also discussed whether oats are toxic or not to celiac patients, and this is an issue that different research groups are trying to figure out.

In this Doctorate Thesis, I studied the participation of oats in the pathogenesis of celiac disease in comparison to the effects of wheat. The role of vegetable oils and proteins of cow's milk in inducing intestinal histopathological changes that occur in the CD was also studied. To this end an experimental laboratory animal model was developed in which the

13

typical intestinal lesions were reproduced by sensitization to the proteins causing the CD and their behavior to the challenges of specific antigens and the exclusion of the toxic components of the diet was studied.

The immunogenic sensitization caused was similar for both avenin and gliadin, further demonstrating cross-reactivity between gliadin and avenins in oats and gluten-challenged animals.

The modification of the type and quality of dietary fat also influenced the severity of intestinal lesions. The use of high quality olive oil shows a protective effect on the intestinal mucosa which reduces edema and inflammatory infiltrate.

The exclusion of cow's milk from the diet also contributed significantly in preventing histological alterations. It is worth noting that these experimental results extrapolated to patients with CD allowed the reversion of the disease symptoms and led to negative results of anti-gliadin, anti-endomysium and even anti-tissue transglutaminase antibodies while consuming gluten.

Our results suggest that cereals may not be the only cause involved in the pathogenesis of celiac disease, but they suggest that other foods frequently consumed could potentiate the sensitization produced by prolamins. In this context, the validation of a sensitization protocol for a reproducible experimental animal model becomes very important and paves the way for future research.

INTRODUCTION

Celiac disease is characterized by a complex symptomatology including growth failure, diarrhea, irritability, vomiting, anorexia, foul-smelling stools, abdominal pain, excessive appetite, rectal prolapse and physical signs such as height and weight below the 25th percentile, muscular atrophy, edema, clubbing, meteorism, recurrent stomatitis, vitamin K deficiency, frequent respiratory infections and pallor (62). In some cases, the disease presents clinical associations with Down syndrome (28), diabetes mellitus (52), dermatitis herpetiformis (44) and neurological disorders such as schizophrenia, epilepsy and intracranial calcifications (19).

The pathogenesis of celiac disease not only involves the toxicity of certain proteins in cereals but also environmental factors. This observation is supported by a mismatch of 30% in identical twins, and 70% amongst HLA-identical siblings. The variability in age at onset between siblings has been attributed to the existence of several symptomatic triggering factors such as diarrhea, pregnancy, surgery and the use of some antibiotics. 10% of first-degree relatives present asymptomatic damage and the association with certain human leukocyte antigens such as HLA-B8, D/DR3, D/DR7, D/Qw2 and D/Q8 (62).

There are other causes that alter the small intestine mucosa and that create a range of differential diagnosis of celiac disease, amongst which we find: gluten intolerance, enteropathy sensitive to cow's milk, intolerance to soy proteins and other transitory food intolerances, gastroenteritis and postgastroenteritis syndromes, giardiasis, autoimmune enteropathy, acquired hypogamaglobulinemia, tropical sprue and protein-energy malnutrition.

The adequate characterization of symptoms and signs of celiac disease in order to achieve a correct diagnosis can be complemented with the detection of immunological markers: antigliadin IgA and IgG antibodies, IgA and IgG anti-endomysial antibodies detected by TIFI and anti-tissue transglutaminase antibodies, which have the effectiveness of anti-endomysium antibodies by means of the methodological application introduced by the quantitative techniques of ELISA. Finally the anatomopathological changes of intestinal mucosal biopsies show increased intraepithelial lymphocytes, inflammatory infiltrate of the lamina propria, macrophage activity and increased cytokine. In addition, the tissue can display full or partial villous atrophy and crypt elongation that were characterized and classified by Marsh (33). This classification is the one used today as the basis for a standardized nomenclature of lesions ranging from grade 0, the preinfiltrative lesion or normal mucosa, grade 1, the infiltrative lesion, characterized by intraepitelial lymphocytosis (more than 30 per 100 enterocytes). The grade 2 lesion, an hyperplasic lesion with an increased crypt depth; the grade 3 lesion (or atrophic) with flattening of the mucosa. The grade 4 lesion is characterized by a hypoplastic mucosa.

History of celiac disease:

100 A.D. Aretaeus of Cappadocia (8) first described celiac diathesis.

1760 Jean Astruc (6) called celiac a particular diarrhea with feces having a milky chyle that could not be absorbed by the intestine.

1888 Samuel Gee (18) described the "celiac disease" in a group of children aged 1-5 years who were undernourished.

1935 Thorwald E. H. Thaysen (53) identified the disease in adults.

1953 WM Dicke (12) noted that with the reduction in wheat consumption during World War II reduced the incidence of "celiac sprue". Later, when the supply of wheat returned to normal, the disease was reintroduced, confirming the importance of this cereal in the genesis of the disease. Together with Van de Kamer, they standardized the diet to treat the disease.

1954 JW Paulley (38) described the characteristic intestinal lesion and associated the disease with the atrophy of the intestinal villi and crypts elongation. He highlighted the exclusion of wheat, barley and rye from the diet as the therapeutic principle to confirm gluten intolerance.

1965 WC McDonald (30) suggested a dominant autosomal inheritance pattern with incomplete penetrance.

1970 GW Meeuwisse (35) implemented the study of three consecutive biopsies for the diagnostic validation of the disease. The first biopsy was applied for the suspected diagnosis, the second was used after the elimination of gluten and the third one after a reintroduction of gluten to confirm its toxicity.

1984-1989 C Ribes-Konickx (45) and TP Chorzelski (15) characterized antigliadin and endomysial antibodies, respectively, both with pathognomonic value.

1991 A great interest comes up in the association with certain HLA antigens (3).

1997 W Dietrich et al. (13) identified part of the transglutaminase enzyme as a component of the chemical structure of anti-endomysium antibodies and as a specific autoantigen of celiac disease therefore closing the circle of the autoimmune pathophysiology of the disease. They emphasized the role of zonulin in the absorption and the increase of intestinal permeability.

Concept of Celiac Disease:

Celiac disease can be defined as a genetic, immune-mediated disease, characterized by the disorder of the proximal small intestinal mucosa associated with a permanent intolerance to gluten that leads to malabsorption syndrome and subsequently to gastrointestinal disease. The elimination of gluten from the diet lead to clinical remission and the normalization of the mucosa (62).

The cereal grains consist essentially of an embryo, located in the center of the seed from which a new plant grows; the endosperm surrounding the embryo and containing the starch reserve and proteins needed for growth; and the episperm, high in fiber, which covers and protects both the embryo and endosperm and which is formed by the aleurone layer, bran and testa. (Figure 1).

The distribution of these components in a wheat grain is illustrated in the following diagram.

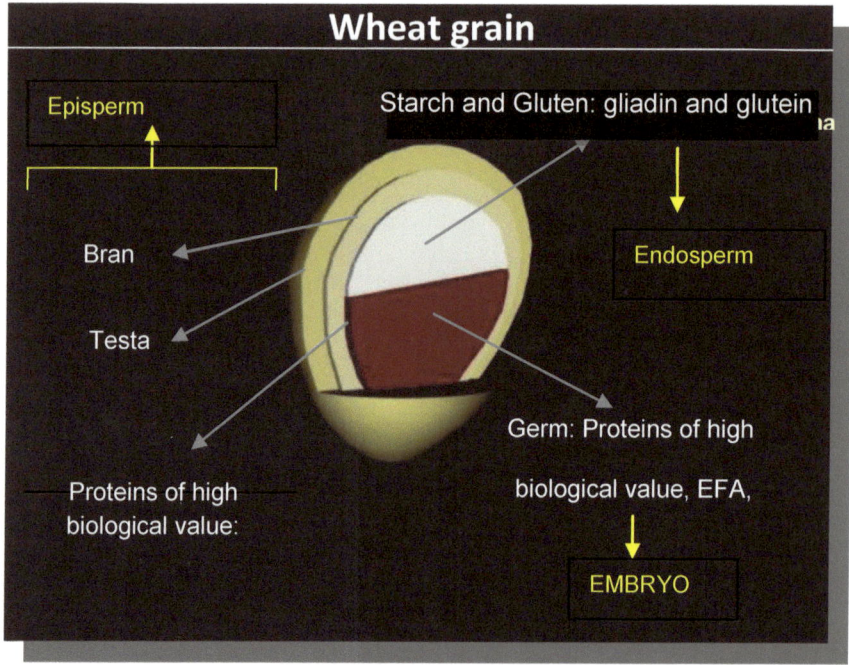

Figure 1. Diagram showing the composition of a wheat grain.

Most of the corn and wheat proteins in the endosperm are glutelins, soluble in alkali and diluted acids, and prolamins, soluble in alcohol solutions (16). The prolamin content is very low in the oats and rice.

Wheat flour is mostly obtained from the endosperm, which consists of 85% gliadin (prolamin) and glutein (glutenin) in an approximate ratio of 1:1 (Figure 2). The toxicity in celiac disease is caused mainly by prolamins. These were identified and characterized by its high content of glutamine and proline and its numerous protein components can be grouped into w-type and g-type while gliadin has an additional a-type. For celiac patients, the toxic fraction of cereals corresponds to the N-terminal domain which has a repeated sequence of amino-acids rich in glutamine, proline and aromatic amino-acids, while the C-terminal domain has a more usual amino-acid composition and no repeated sequence (63, 64). Charbonier et al. (9) particularly related the toxicity to the alpha and beta-gliadins and other peptides with molecular weights between 5 and 10,000 daltons. These proteins, constituted by different molecular species have special properties that allow the formation of an elastic, compact mass when mixed with water. This mass called gluten is characterized by high contents of glutamine and proline.

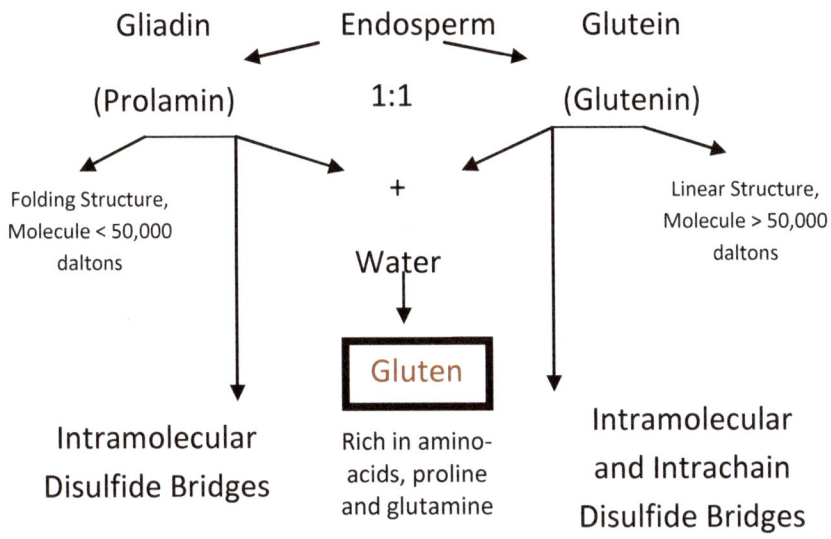

Figure 2. Protein composition of the endosperm.

Gluten polypeptide chains lack helical structure, probably due to proline, the amino-acid that prevents the formation of this type of structure.

Glutenin is a linear association of polypeptide chains with a molecular weight between 20,000 and 100,000 daltons (24) .The subunits ared linked together by disulfide bridges that result in polymers of high molecular weight, from 50,000 to several million daltons.

Gliadins consist of relatively small uniform units with folding structures maintained by disulfide bridges. The molecular weights of gliadin molecules vary between 16,000 and 50,000 daltons. Among other things, the disulfide bridges have an influence on the extractability of different gluten protein fractions (65). Gliadin hydration favors the formation of a viscous, fluid, extensible but inelastic mass and, in fact, determines the final volume of wheat flour bread.

In oats, the main protein is avenin, which can be extracted in ethyl alcohol thanks to its solubility.

Corn is formed by prolamin, zein and glutelin, a mixture of different molecular weight proteins linked together by disulfide bridges forming complexes that significantly alter the grinding process (16).

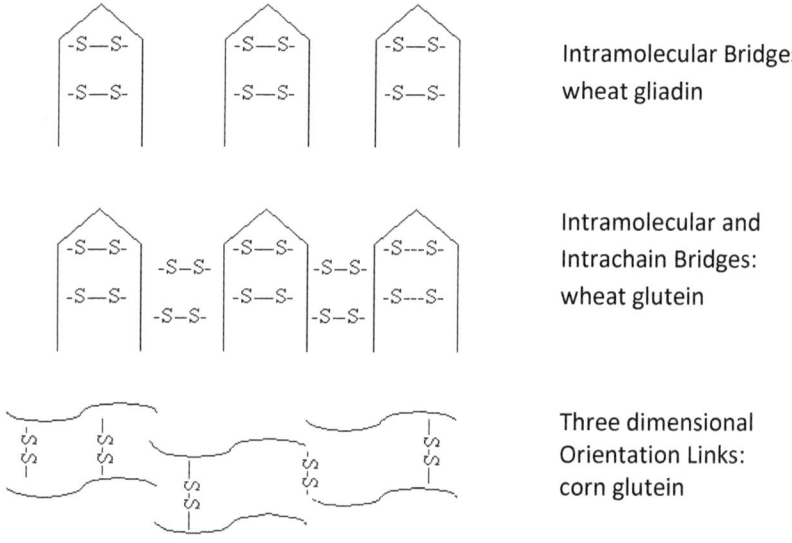

Intramolecular Bridges: wheat gliadin

Intramolecular and Intrachain Bridges: wheat glutein

Three dimensional Orientation Links: corn glutein

Figure 3. Disulfide bridges in cereal proteins.

The prolamins of wheat, barley and rye have groups with high structural homology. While oats have been regarded for years as one of these cereals with toxic components, their participation in the pathogenesis of celiac disease was questioned by some authors (22, 46, 55, 51, 23). The pathogenesis of celiac disease has been extensively studied, but there are still many questions which remain unsolved and finding an answer to them is critical to developing a specific treatment. For this reason the use of experimental models is very important since they enable a better understanding of the behavior of the intestinal mucosa when challenged to immunogenic proteins and of the modifications can be made to the immune status in the target organs of these animals. To this end, we consider important to investigate the cellular basis of the small intestine of mice subjected to adequate immunization against proteins inducing cereals celiac disease and its response to challenges with proteins under study.

Characteristics of the absorptive surface of the intestine:

Under normal conditions, the digestive tract experiences a constant process of maturation, differentiation and remodeling of the mucosa. In the case of the small intestine, the mucosa is formed by a coating of epithelial cells and underlying connective tissue which together make up the villi or digitiform protrusions of the lamina propria. This, in turn, includes the basement membrane, synthesized by enterocytes and myofibroblasts, the extracellular matrix and the connective tissue cells. It also contains cells of the autonomic nervous system and its extensions, smooth muscle cells and local immune system cells, vascular elements and other cells that reside there only temporarily (61). The mucosa is occupied by simple tubular glands whose cul-de-sac reaches the muscularis mucosa which they normally never perforate. These are called glands or crypts of Lieberkühn.

Epithelium:

The epithelium is simple and columnar in shape; it covers the free edge of the villi and the surface of the intervillous spaces. It is composed of:

- Absorption surface cells: these are the most abundant cells in epithelium; about 25 µm in length with oval nuclei located at the basal pole. Its apical surface exhibits a brush border with microvilli of approximately 1 µm in length and whose free surface is covered by a layer of glycocalyx. These elements form a continuous narrow strip called striated border. The cells reesterify the fatty acids in triglycerides, form chylomicrons and carry most of the nutrients absorbed into the lamina propria for distribution to the rest of the body (17). The layer of glycocalyx not only protects microvilli against autodigestion, but their enzyme components participate in the terminal digestion of disaccharides and dipeptides releasing their monomers.

The lateral cell membranes of these cells have complex intercellular junctions formed by narrow or tight junctions (*zonula ocludens*), adherens junctions (*zonula adherens*), desmosomes and gap junctions (nexus or gap) which seal with adjacent cells. Tight junctions prevent the passage of circulating material in the intestinal lumen into the lamina propria of the intenstines via paracellular transport or from the lamina propia into the lumen. The different intercellular junctions of the intestinal epithelium are illustrated in the scheme and electron micrograph reproduced below (Figures 4 and 5).

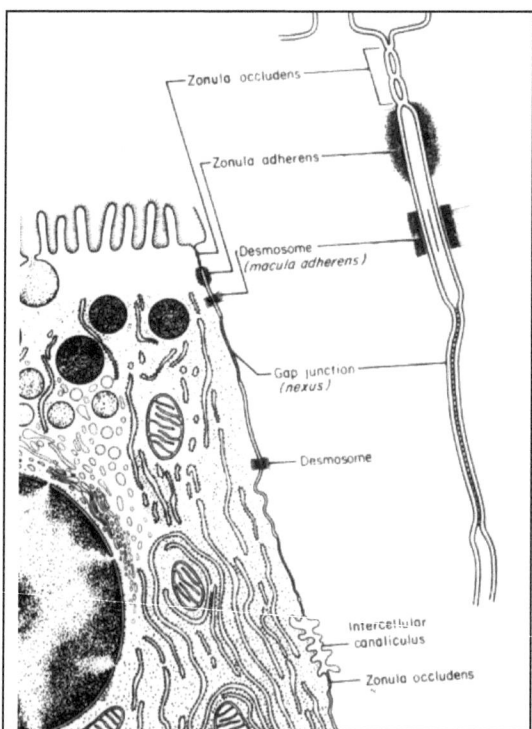

Figure 4. Scheme of intercellular junctions of epithelial cells taken from Don W. Fawcett, A Textbook of Histology Chapman and Hall New York-London 1994.

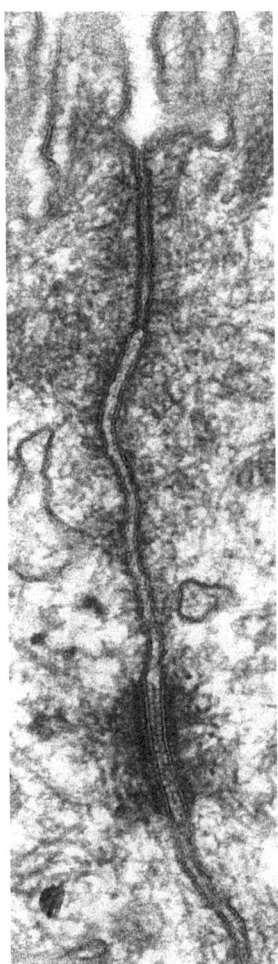

Figure 5. Microphotograph of junction complexes between two enterocytes, kindly provided by Dr. Amalia Passoli, Rockefeller University, and published in Cell (39). Reproduced with editorial permission.

- Goblet cells: unicellular glands that produce mucinogen, whose hydrated form is mucin, a component of mucus that constitutes a protective layer on the luminal surface of the intestinal mucosa.
- Enteroendocrine cells: they are pyramidal in shape and have a narrow apex and widened basal pole. Dense secretory granules containing the synthesized hormone products are detected in the cytoplasmic matrix. These cells produce serotonin, secretin, cholecystokinin and glucagon-like substance. They also produce somatotrofina and endorphin.

- Paneth cells: they are located at the bottom of the crypts of Lieberkühn and produce lysozyme, a bactericidal enzyme that disrupts the bacteria walls.
- M cells: they have been assimilated into the mononuclear phagocyte system; they are modified enterocytes in areas of lymph nodes.
- Stem cells: they are divided into different groups: absorbent, goblet, enteroendocrine and Paneth. They have intense mitotic activity and proliferate to repopulate the crypt epithelium, and mucosal surface and villous.

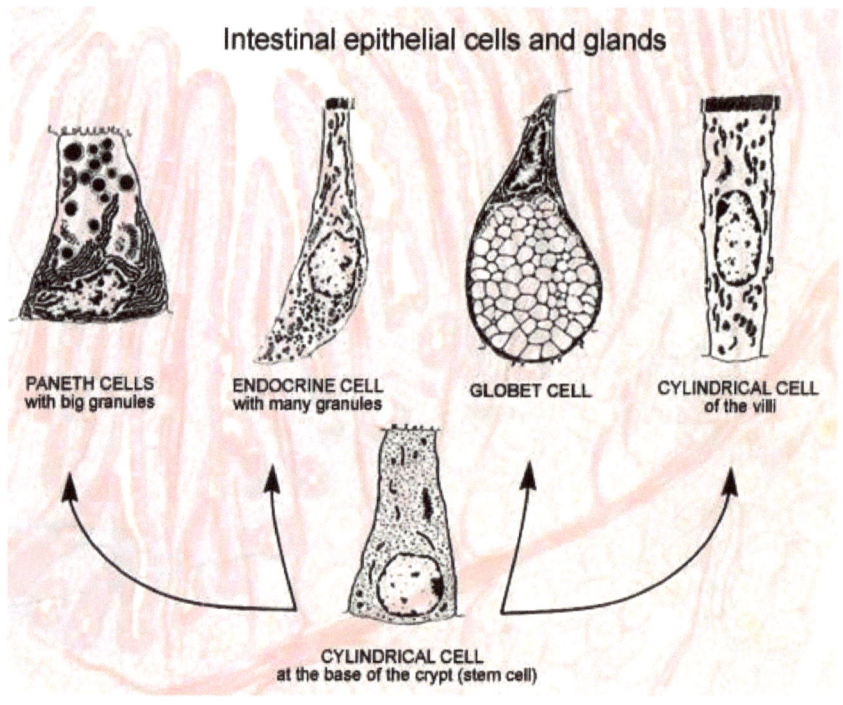

Figure 6. Scheme of intestinal epithelial cells taken (and modified) from the Tratado de Histología de Ham, A. W. y Cormack D. H. Octava Edición. 1983. Editorial Interamericana. Mexico DF

Basement membrane:

It is the interface between the epithelium and the connective matrix. It is a thin laminar structure immediately below the epithelium, which allows the fixation to the underlying connective tissue. In the small intestine, this is a structure of about 100 nm in thickness separated from the enterocytes by an electrolucid space of about 20 nm, which outlines the contour of the epithelial cells base.

It is now accepted that during the transit of chylomicrons from enterocytes into the lamina propria there are gaps in their continuity. The absence of gaps during fasting suggests that they are temporary and a demonstration that the basement membrane responds to functional requirements (42).

Immunopathology in celiac disease:

the immunological abnormalities characteristic of the celiac disease include an increase in the circulating antibodies, intraepithelial lymphocyte infiltrate and infiltrate in the lamina propria of IgG, A and M plasma cells, mast cells, eosinophils and T cells (TC). The CD4 TCs dominate this compartment. Eosinophils produce cytokines such as IL-5 which contribute to the synthesis of IgA. There is macrophage activation and local increase in the production of cytokines, such as the tumor necrosis factor.

The amino-acid residue resistant to protease would act as intestinal T cells epitopes. The increased activity of the tissue transglutaminase (tTG) in the duodenal mucosa of celiac patients, together with the discovery of gliadin as the preferred substrate of this enzyme, suggests that it plays a pivotal role in the development of the disease. Being a protein rich in amide groups, gliadin is a substrate of tTG and in the CD, the conjugate formed by both molecules during gliadin deamidation creates new epitopes with increased affinity for HLA DQ2 or DQ8 antigen, and a potentiation of gluten-specific T cells. The binding of these deamidated residual peptides via tTG with peptide-sensitized CD4 TL produces significant quantities of cytokines with the subsequente cytotoxicity for epithelial cell. These reactions cause the appearance of anti-gliadin, anti-endomysium and anti-tissue transglutaminase (32) antibodies.

Lymphocytes present in the intestinal tract account for up to 20% of the body's total lymphocytes and are divided into different groups: lymphoid follicles, intraepithelial lymphocytes and lamina propria lymphocytes.

The antigen-presenting cells produce mediators that induce T cells to differentiate into T1 and T2 and cause macrophage activation, delayed hypersensitivity, and allergic response.

The antigen reacts directly with the immunoglobulins in the B cells membrane; subsequently , the antigen is internalized, fragmented, and associated to the HLA II, and expressed on the membrane of the B cells (Figure 7). Then, if the antigen finds the right stimulus of a CD4 cell, the production of immunoglobulins can be created. Collaboration between B cells and CD4 occurs when both cells contact and due to the presence of HLA II and the antigen as well as the release of lymphokines. Antigens may be taken up by macrophages that act as antigen-presenting cells and that together with B cells are expressed on the B cells HLA II membrane.

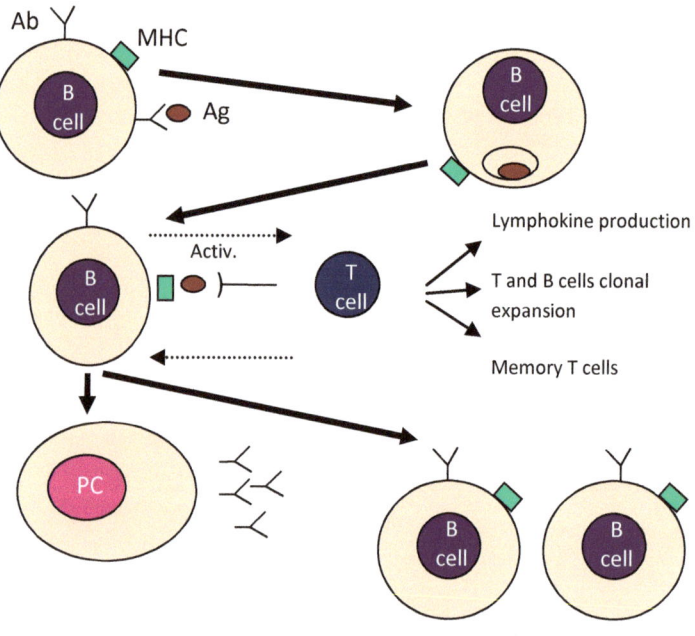

Figure 7. Scheme of the immunological changes that occur in celiac disease.

Evidence that the HLA DQ2 molecule is expressed by more than 90% of individuals with celiac disease versus 21% in the general population suggests that genetic factors are important in the development of celiac disease. In a minority of patients, this is associated with the HLA DQ8 (60).

Celiac disease can be considered an inflammatory disorder mediated by T cells with autoimmune features. Most of the gluten epitopes that are recognized by T cells are specific glutamine residues that have been converted to glutamic acid. This deamidation is mediated by the tissue transglutaminase enzyme, the main endomysial autoantigen in the disease (49).

Interleukin 15 induces the enterocytes apoptosis in samples of untreated celiac patients and participates in the modulation of epithelial changes in celiac disease, indicating that cytokines have an unexpected role in the pathological manifestations of celiac disease (29).

An accessible animal model should be of upmost importance to investigate the pathogenesis and treatment of celiac disease as highlighted by Troncone and Ferguson (58) in their experimental study. In this research, systemic immunization with gliadin was performed to achieve a mouse model of gluten-induced enteropathy. These researchers observed no changes in the jejunal mucosa of BALB mice that were fed with a diet containing gluten after being parenterally immunized with gliadin and complete Freund's adjuvant. They detected mucosal changes with the presence of additional factors such as intestinal anaphylaxis by infection with the parasite *Nippostrongylus brasiliensis* or after a graft versus host reaction. Thus they suggested that the increased permeability of the intestinal mucosa would be critical and that gliadin may not be a sufficient condition to develop a T cells mediated intestinal lesion.

Maurano et al. (34) also used parenteral immunization with gliadin. They tried to induce tolerance reducing the expression of immune response to wheat gliadin in mice by intranasal administration of the alpha gliadin.

An animal model of gluten-sensitive enteropathy should present an injury of the intestinal mucosa characterized by shortening of the villi, crypt hyperplasia, infiltrate of lymphocytes and other inflammatory cells in the epithelium and lamina propria.

Histopathology in celiac disease:

One of the parameter that is altered early in celiac disease are intraepithelial lymphocytes (IELs) located next to the basement membrane and with a normal density of 20-40/100 epithelial cells. In celiac disease, the IELs density increases significantly (>40/100 epithelial cells), the IELs are often larger and move toward the apical pole of the intestinal villi (56).

Comparable morphological changes have also been described in cow's milk intolerance enteropathy and in other causes of lesion to the intestinal mucosa in childhood (36).

The gastrointestinal tract has both immunological and non-immunological defense mechanisms that intervene in the barriers for absorption of macromolecules. Secretory IgA is an immunoglobulin which is produced in greater amounts in the intestine and that has the ability to bind proteins to form large protein complexes, thus avoiding absorption. Two percent of the molecules that are absorbed intact would create oral tolerance. Both the systemic and local immune system are responsible for developing oral tolerance when the antigens pass through the intestinal wall barrier formed by epithelial cells, the glycocalyx and its enzymes.

Hypersensitivity to food is the result of the loss or absence of tolerance and its etiology is multifactorial. When immunity occurs with tissue damage it is called allergy or hypersensitivity. One of the most allergenic food components are cow's milk proteins, and there are over 40 proteins which can generate an allergic response. Of these the most common are: heat-labile protein (bovine serum albumin, alpha-globulins, alpha-lactalbumin) and heat-resistant proteins such as casein and beta-lactoglobulin.

The presence of tight junctions in the apical border of intestinal epithelial cells block the intercellular transport, which means the absorption of intestinal contents must penetrate the plasma membrane in the brush border, incorporate into the apical cytoplasm and permeate the lateral cell membrane permeate to access the basolateral spaces of epithclial cells. The lateral plasma membranes of adjacent cells are separated in the basal region of the epithelium and it is in these intercellular spaces where chylomicrons accumulate during the transportation process.

The plasma membrane at the cell base is in close contact with a continuous basal lamina which closes the space and limits the basal portion of the epithelium. The absorbed and accumulated materials must pass through this barrier to reach the capillaries and lymphatic vessels of the intestinal villi.

The postprandial state has sparked renewed interest since it was discovered that triglyceride-rich lipoproteins are involved in the development of atherosclerosis. For this reason, many researchers have focused their studies on the analysis of lipoprotein metabolism in response to a standardized fat diet. Hennig et al. (21) found that the serum from hypertriglyceridemic patients alters the permeability of the endothelial barrier. Other studies have described a decline in cell viability after incubation of muscle cells with chylomicron remnants (66). These results raised the question of whether the fat transport speed through the intestinal epithelium varies with the type and quality of the fats and whether a slowdown in the transport of chylomicrons may contribute to the alteration of the intestinal architecture.

In disorders with structural abnormality of the mucosa, the process of cell migration from crypts bases to the ends of the villi can be accelerated and immature cells tend to reach the apex of the villi and presumably be less able to process dietary fat (60).

In a polarized secretory cell, the Golgi complex has a single large dictyosomes that occupies an intermediate position between the nucleus and the cell surface where the discharge is produced. Golgi complexes with these characteristics are observed, for example, in cells in the intestinal mucosa, the thyroid gland and the exocrine pancreas (11). It should consider whether resynthesized triglycerides in the smooth endoplasmic reticulum, which continue their path through the cell cytoplasm to be packaged as chylomicrons in the Golgi complex, play a role in the lesions produced due to malabsorption pathologies, since in normal conditions 95% of dietary fats are incorporated in the intestine. In connection with this observation, it should be noted that it is not uncommon to find a relation between diseases involving the intestine and pancreas, such as diabetes and celiac disease, or diabetes and allergy to cow's milk proteins. It is also possible to find a relation between thyroid disease and enteropathy, such as in the case of patients with food allergy and hypothyroidism.

At present, it has been proven that the consumption of fish oil decreases triglyceride concentration in blood plasma. An interesting fact is that Denmark, the main producer of fish oil in the European Union and also a major importer, is one of the countries with the lowest seroprevalence of celiac disease, 1:500 compared with 1:100 or 1:50 in other regions (32).

It is currently accepted that inflammatory changes similar to those ocurring in celiac disease can also be seen in cow's milk intolerance (36). The proteins in cow's milk and wheat are globular macromolecules without intermolecular crosslinks. Both types of proteins have intrachain disulfide bridges in their molecular structure and the adverse reactions to these foods manifest in common signs and symptoms. Typically, the mucosa in the enteropathy sensitive to cow's milk is characterized by its thinness (31). Pathological changes frequently occur in patches (32). There is an increase in the intraepithelial lymphocyte count, although not to the level found in celiac disease (41); also, dense accumulations of fat were observed in the epithelium (60). These observations made it reasonable to think of allergy to cow's milk proteins as a trigger for celiac disease and the importance of studying the changes that the inclusion or exclusion of milk could create in an animal model sensitized to wheat proteins was evaluated.

The high prevalence of celiac disease, together with the difficulty in following the diet requiered by the treatment, makes further research it very important in order to better understand the mechanisms involved in this pathology. For this, it is required an accessible animal model and an easy reproduction protocol, which are the main contributions intended for this research.

Once the experimental model is obtained, it will be possible to rethink the role that wheat has held for many years in the development of the disease, and to analyze the role that other elements of the diet can have as triggers or mitigating factors.

OBJECTIVES

GENERAL OBJECTIVES

To establish an experimental model of celiac disease in laboratory animals and study the histopathological changes in the intestine.

To determine the participation of oats and other molecules different from cereal prolamins in the pathogenesis of this disease.

SPECIFIC OBJECTIVES

To develop in laboratory animals and adequate gluten sensitization so they become intolerant to that protein and to assess the histopathological changes of the experimental enteropathy to achieve the standardization of the procedure and the reliability thereof.

To compare the intestinal morphology after a challenge with gluten and oats in animals immunized with gliadin or avenin and to check the presence of crossed immunoreactivity between both proteins.

To analyze the histopathologic differences in models sensitized to wheat modifying dietary fat.

To determine whether the inclusion or exclusion of cow's milk in the challenge diet of animals immunized with gliadin causes changes at intestinal level indicative of the role it plays in the pathogenesis of the disease.

MATERIALS AND METHODS

Experimental animals:

Young, adult, BALB female and male mice were used, weighing approximately 25 to 30 grams, bred in our animal facility under controlled conditions of light (14 hours of light and 10 hours of darkness) and temperature (23°C ± 3°C).

Female mice were mated with males of proven fertility during 12 hours. Once the pregnancy was confirmed, the females received a gluten-free diet. For this purpose the commercial feed for the mice was replaced with food developed in our laboratory. This diet was continued after the birth of offspring and throughout lactation. Once produced weaning, the calves had access to it only gluten-free diet provided to mothers, and for a period of six weeks prior to immunological sensitization.

Diet compositions:

Gluten-free diet:

This base gluten-free diet was prepared with the following components:

Corn Nestum	250 g.
Rice Nestum	250 g.

Soy milk	350 g.
Cow's milk (skim powdered)	150 g.
Sunflower seeds (peeled)	750 g.
Sunflower oil	250 cc.

Challenge diets:

Oats enriched diet: corn and rice Nestum were replaced by equal amounts of oats.

Gluten enriched diet: corn and rice Nestum were replaced by equal amounts of whole wheat.

Gluten/extra-virgin olive oil enriched diet: the previous base was used but the sunflower oil was replaced with a mixture of equal parts of extra-virgin olive oil and fish oil.

Gluten/low quality olive oil enriched diet: the previous base was used but the sunflower oil was replaced by equal amounts of commercial olive oil of low quality.

Gluten/low quality olive oil enriched diet with exclusion of milk: similar to the above diet but with the exclusion of milk.

The nutritional values of the dietary components are detailed in Figure 8.

The mixtures were kept refrigerated as dry powder: water and oil were added to the preparation at the moment of preparing the cookies to knead. Squares of approximately 3 cm were cut, which were placed in a tray and cooked in a microwave at 160° until dehydration.

The cookies were placed in the feeding dishes of the mice cages.

	Kcal	Fat (g)	Carbs (g)	Proteins (g)
Corn Nestum	370	1.1	85	5.4
Rice Nestum	370	0.5	85	5.6
Soy milk *	523	31	52.8	14.2
Cow's milk **	359	1.2	51.7	35.3
Sunflower seeds***	630	70		30
Sunflower oil	900	100		
Whole wheat	340	70	2	16
Oats	383		31	13.3

* Rich in linoleic acid, linolenic acid and lysine amino-acids.
** Skim powdered.
*** Peeled. Rich in palmitic, stearic, oleic and linoleic acids and essential amino-acids such as isoleucine and tryptophan.

Figure 8. Nutrition information per a 100 g diet.

Experimental models

Immune sensitization to gliadin and avenin

For the immune sensitization to gliadin and avenin, the technique described by Troncone and Ferguson (58) was applied, following the protocol described below:

Mice 6 weeks after weaning were treated with:

- Subcutaneous injection on the back of the animals of an emulsion of 50 µg of wheat gliadin (Sigma) or avenin (obtained by alcoholic extraction) emulsified with 50 µg of Freund's adjuvant.
- Repetition of the emulsion injection within 15 days of the first application.

During the sensitization period, the animals continued the gluten-free diet which was used until the start of the experimental treatments within 15 days after the last injection.

Alcoholic extraction of avenin

- Place 0.125 g of ground oat flour in a 10 mL propylene tube.
- Add 5 ml of 60% ethanol solution and incubate for 1 hour at room temperature on a rotary shaker at 750 rpm.
- Centrifuge at 3500 rpm for 10 minutes.
- Transfer the supernatant-avenin to clean 10 mL propylene tubes and apply freeze-drying.

Preparation of the emulsion: suitable amounts of gliadin or avenin were weighed and suspended in Freund's adjuvant (Sigma) to obtain a final concentration of 50 μg/50 μl.

(The general protocol for obtaining avenin was kindly provided by Dr. Enrique Mendez, personal communication).

Challenge with gluten or oats:

As of 15 days after the last sensitizing injection, the mice were divided into 6 groups of 6 animals each and subjected to the following treatments:

Group 1: gliadin-sensitized mice challenged with gluten enriched diet.

Group 2: gliadin-sensitized mice challenged with oats-containing diet.

Group 3: avenin-sensitized mice challenged with gluten enriched diet.

Group 4: avenin-sensitized mice challenged with oats enriched diet.

Group 5: gliadin-sensitized control mice with gluten-free diet.

Group 6: avenin-sensitized control mice with gluten-free diet.

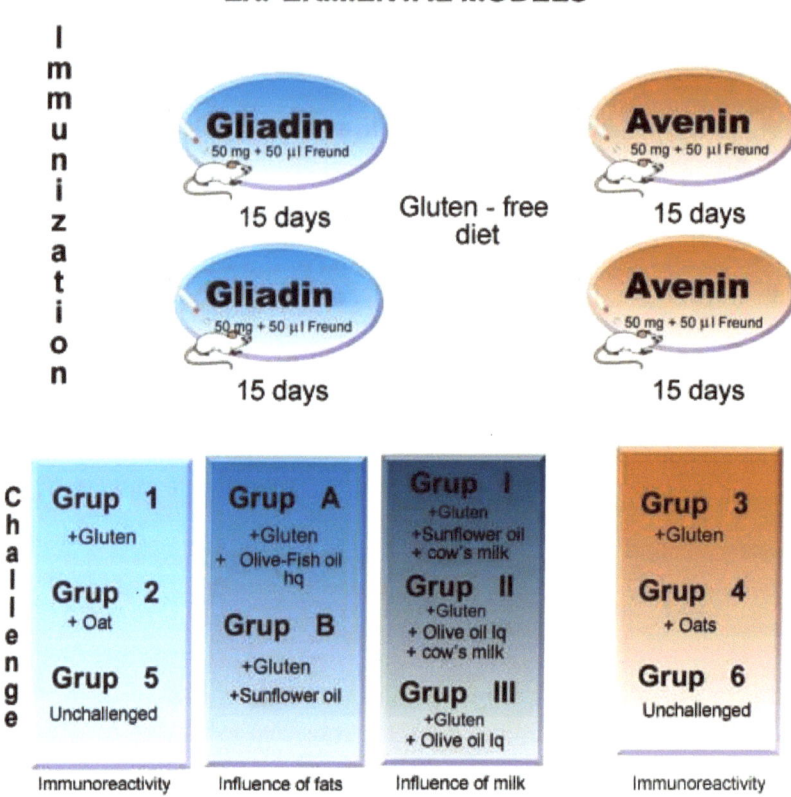

Figure 9. Scheme of the immune sensitization to gliadin and avenin protocol. (hq: high quality, lq: low quality).

<u>Challenge with gluten replacing the type and quality of dietary lipids:</u>

The aim was to evaluate the influence of the type and quality of dietary fats in 6 gliadin-sensitized mice fed with diets containing different types of fats. The immunologically sensitized mice were divided into two groups and challenged as follows:

Group A: three gliadin-sensitized mice received a gluten enriched diet with a mixture of equal parts of extra virgin olive oil (with free acidity expressed in oleic acid of less than 11g%) and fish oil as fat intake.

Group B: three mice were challenged with a gluten enriched diet with sunflower oil.

Challenge with gluten incorporating and excluding cow's milk:

Six gliadin-immunologically sensitized mice were used and divided into three groups and subjected to the following challenges:

Group I: two animals were challenged with gluten and fed with the standardized amounts of sunflower oil and cow's milk.

Group II: two animals were challenged with gluten; the diet included low quality olive oil and the standardized amount of cow's milk.

Group III: two animals were challenged with gluten and low quality olive oil, excluding cow's milk from the diet.

Morphological Studies:

In all the experimental models, morphological studies of the small intestine were performed 7 and 21 days after the conclusion of the treatment. Mice were anesthetized maintaining their conditions in accordance with the Guidelines for the handling and training of laboratory animals published by the Universities Federation for Animal Welfare and the Local Institutional Animal Care Committee, which are in line with international regulations. Using exploratory laparotomy, the proximal small intestine was fixed and samples which were subsequently processed for analysis were taken.

Light microscopy: tissue samples were fixed in 4% buffered formalin in phosphate buffer preparation, pH 7.4, dehydrated in increasing concentrations of ethyl alcohol, cleared in xylene and embedded in paraffin. Five micron sections were stained with hematoxylin-eosin.

Electron microscopy: segments of intestine were fixed in Karnovsky's mixture using the following components: 1.5% glutaraldehyde, 1.5% formaldehyde in 0.1 M cacodylate buffer, pH 7.4. Then the samples were postfixed in 1% osmium tetroxide, dehydrated in increasing concentrations of acetone and embedded in epoxy resin (Araldite).

Slices of 0,5-1 μm were obtained and stained with 1% toluidine blue (TB) in 1% borax in order to observe them under high resolution photonic microscopy. The ultra-thin sections (80 nm) were cut on an JUM-7 ultramicrotome (JEOL) equipped with diamond knives mounted on nickel grids and contrasted with uranyl acetate and lead citrate. Observations were recorded on a ZEISS LEO-906 electron microscope.

Intestine sections immersed in paraffin and stained with hematoxylin-eosin made it possible to examine the complete cross sections of intestine at different levels of the samples and to comprehensively evaluate the histopathological changes in various animal models The semi-thin sections of material immersed in Araldite and stained with toluidine blue allow the observation with greater resolution and the record of changes in digital photographs.

In selected groups, morphometric measurements of the height between the apex of the villi and the depth of the crypts were made. The values were expressed in microns.

Morphological alterations were studied by light microscopy in all cases and in more representative models by electron microscopy.

Statistic analysis:

In models challenged with gluten replacing the type and quality of dietary lipids (n = 6), the histopathological consequences of modifying the oils in the challenge diet were analyzed using morphometric data obtained from micrographs of tissue samples using the software Motic Images Plus 2.0.

Six mice were subdivided into two groups and three study variables were considered: a) height of villi, b) base width and c) intestinal mucosa thickness. The data obtained from each group were averaged for each of the variables. For statistical analysis, the software SigmaStat 3.1 was used to determine the mean, standard deviation (SD) and significance level.

Clinical cases:

Ten pediatric patients with symptoms and positive celiac serology were treated at the medical center Sanatorio Allende, Córdoba. They underwent a clinical examination, anthropometry and laboratory determinations. The tests included lab tests for anti-gliadin antibodies (AG), anti-endomysium antibodies (AE) and anti-tissue transglutaminase antibodies in some patients (performed by Dr. Silvia Barzón). Before assessing the need for an intestinal biopsy, patients voluntarily followed a strict diet excluding cow's milk, goat's milk and soy milk and their derivatives for two months.

All patients received supplemental calcium and vitamin D. Patients continued to consume gluten. They were allowed to eat beef once a week and were instructed to decrease the amount of sunflower oil in their diets and to incorporate extra virgin olive oil. Once the diet was completed, they underwent a clinical examination and antibody serum dosage. The results of gliadin antibodies (QUANTA LiteTM Celiac DGP Screen, INOVA Diagnostics, USA) were considered positive when titers obtained by ELISA were higher than 20 AU. Endomysial antibodies were measured by indirect immunofluorescence using a commercial kit (IMMCO Diagnostics system, USA).

RESULTS

Normal morphology of the intestinal epithelium:

Unimmunized animals fed the the gluten-free diet, have an intestinal mucosa with leaf-like digitiform villi, lined with simple columnar epithelium with irregular borders. The elongated nuclei are located basally. Two cell types are recognized, enterocytes and goblet cells. The central axis shows reduced thickness and is formed by a complex connective tissue that is the extension of the lamina propria (Fig. 10).

At higher magnification, it is possible to see a well-defined striated border of equal thickness and homogeneous along the whole epithelium on the apical area.

The examination of the intestinal epithelium by electron microscopy allows the visualization of the ultrastructural characteristics of highly polarized absorptive cells (Fig. 11a). The plasma membrane delimiting these cells shows different specializations in its faces. The apical surface has numerous parallel microvilli uniformly sized, of approximately 1.5 microns in length. From the ends of microvilli, branched filaments emerge which interdigitate to form a cover or glycocalyx. Microvilli have a frame of longitudinal microfilaments that extend from the base into the terminal web in the apical region of the cell. The sides form juxtaluminal junction complexes and develop folds that interdigitate with those of the adjacent cells.

In the basal area, the plasma membrane is supported on a basal lamina under which cells of the lamina propria, blood vessels and lymph vessels are observed.

The enterocyte nuclei located basally have an oval profile, with peripheral heterochromatin surrounding the abundant euchromatin.

In the cytoplasm, a very well-developed system of endomembrane is observed. In the apical area, numerous tubules and cisterns of the smooth endoplasmic reticulum as well as numerous elongated mitochondria are observed. In the supranuclear area, we can find the Golgi complex, free ribosomes and rough endoplasmic reticulum parallel cisterns lateral to the Golgi complex. In the perinuclear area, we can see lipid droplets with varying degrees of processing, coalescing in vacuoles that acquire different outlines (Fig. 11 b and c).

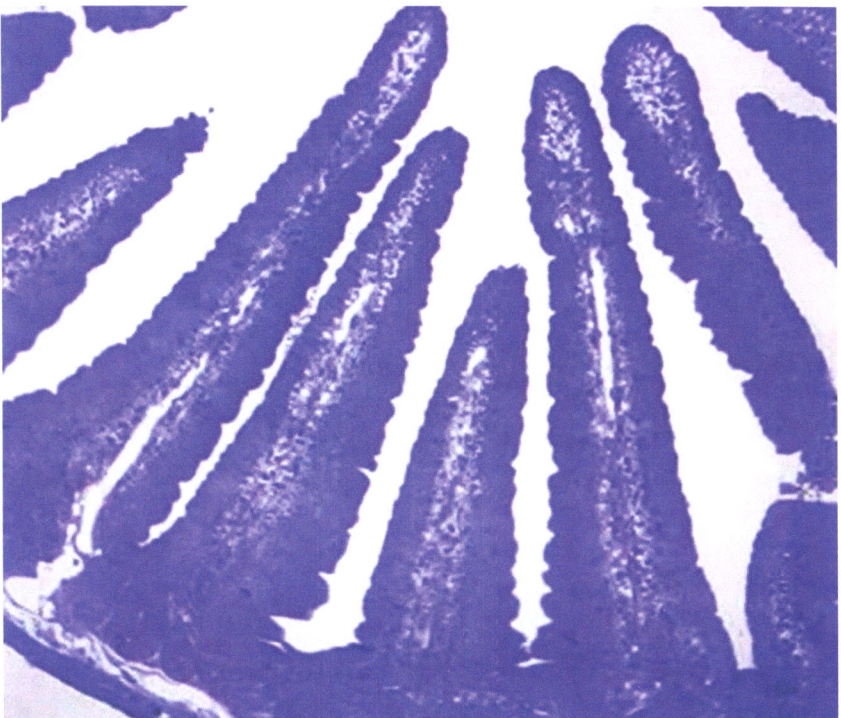

Figure 10. Microphotograph of a cross section of proximal small intestine of a mouse with digitiform villi and irregular borders. Most lining cells are absorptive and have a striated border. Numerous intensely stained nuclei are observed in the connective tissue axis. Araldite. TB.

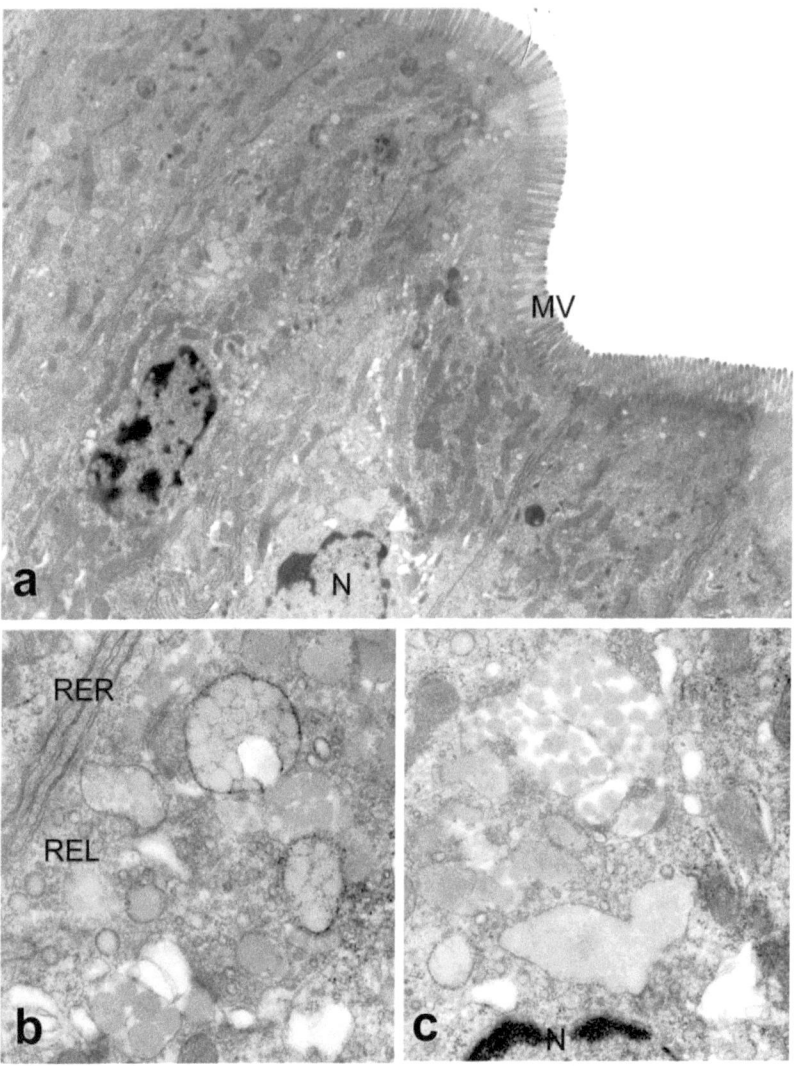

Figure 11. Electron micrographs of a normal mouse intestinal epithelium. a: Microvilli (MV) are observed in the apical surface and the elongated nuclei (N) in the basal area. The cytoplasm has abundant endoplasmic reticulum and mitochondria, Golgi complexes and perinuclear lipid vacuoles. Magnification: 4,500 X. b: Cytoplasm of enterocytes with smooth endoplasmic reticulum (SER) cisterns, rough endoplasmic reticulum (RER) and lipid vacuoles of different density and different levels of processing. Lipid micelles are incorporated into the membranes. c: Near a nucleus (N), coalescing lipid droplets can be seen adopting different profiles. b and c: Magnification: 21,500 X.

Intestinal immune reactivity to gliadin and avenin:

Control animals:

Cross sections of proximal small intestine were analyzed in two groups of 6 animals: mice immunized with gliadin or avenin, which continued to be fed with the gluten-free diet.

These control animals exhibit intestinal villi with a morphological organization compatible with that described for normal animals (Fig. 12 and 13).

Animals challenged with gluten or oats:

Two groups of 6 gliadin-immunologically sensitized animals and challenged with gluten or oats and two groups of 6 animals injected with avenin and subjected to the same challenge previously mentioned were histologically studied. Biopsies were performed on days 7 and 21 of the challenge diets.

In the intestinal mucosa of all animals, inflammatory infiltrate can be seen.

The challenge with both proteins make the villi have a less scalloped outline, which acquire a conical shape with wider bases and present an increase in the diameter of the connective tissue axis, due to edema and cellular infiltrate (Fig. 14 to 17).

The adjuvant-enhanced antigen injection was effective to sensitize the mice and achieve an adequate parenteral immunization to gliadin and avenin.

The morphological alterations were more evident when a challenge was performed with the protein opposite to that used for sensitization (Fig. 15 and 17).

Similar changes are observed in the samples taken on days 7 and 21.

When analyzing the images obtained from the intestine sections of 36 mice in the first stage of the research, it was found that studying the role of oats did not require morphometry as histopathological changes are very significant in the 24 animals challenged.

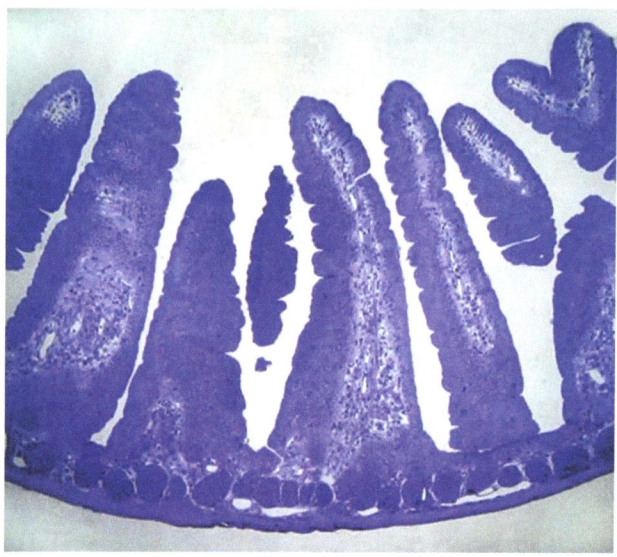

Figure 12. Cross section of the intestine of a control animal immunized with gliadin. The villi maintain their digitiform appearance and irregular borders. Araldite. TB.

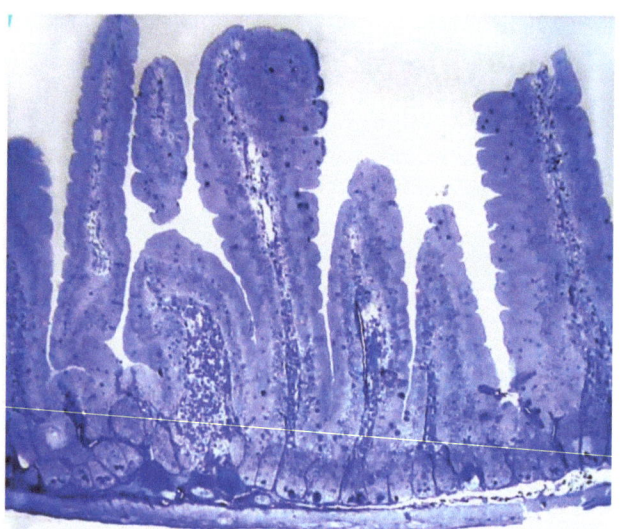

Figure 13. Intestinal mucosa of an avenin-injected control animal. The villi have a normal appearance. Araldite. TB.

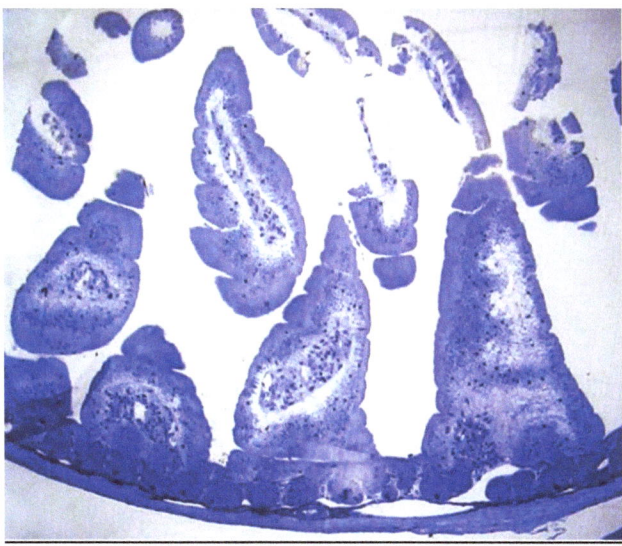

Figure 14. Intestine of an animal injected with gliadin and challenged with gluten for 7 days. Conical villi, edema and inflammatory infiltrate in the lamina propria are observed. Araldite. TB.

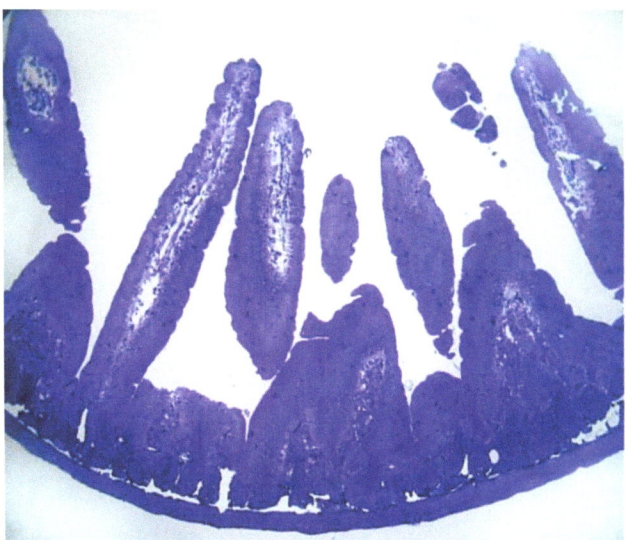

Figure 15. Cross section of intestinal mucosa of an animal immunized with gliadin and challenged with oats for 7 days. Most villi lose their digitiform shape and have wide bases. Araldite. TB

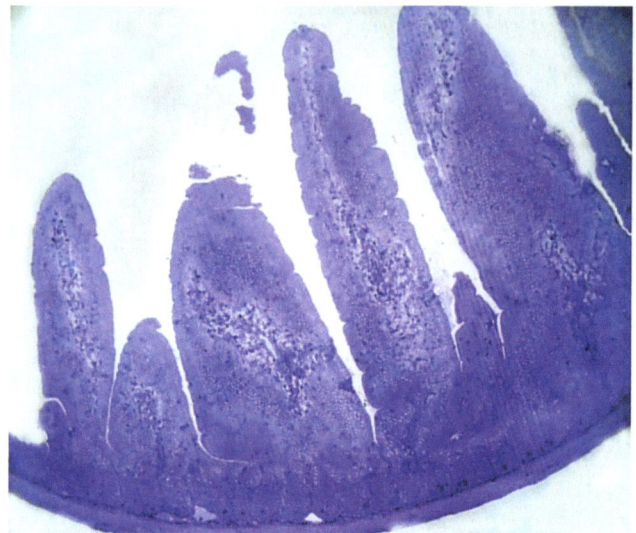

Figure 16. Intestinal mucosa of an animal injected with avenin and challenged with oats for 7 days. Some villi have wider bases and the connective tissue axis presents inflammatory infiltrate. Araldite. TB.

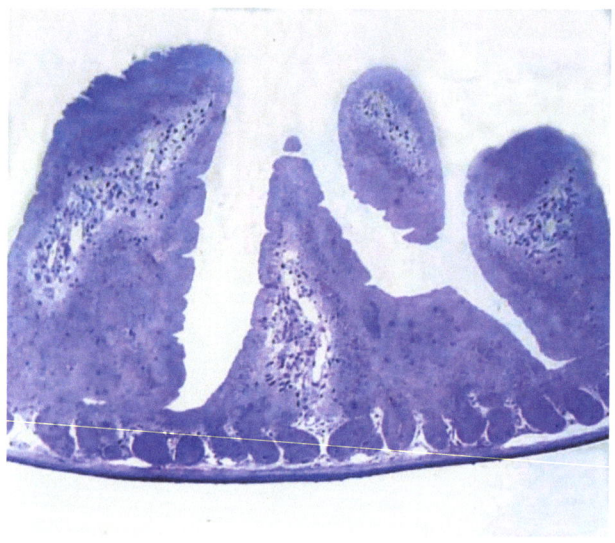

Figure 17. Proximal intestine of an animal immunized with avenin and challenged with gluten for 7 days. Widened-base, shorter, reduced villi per field are observed. Araldite. TB.

Influence of dietary fat:

In order to analyze the influence of different types of dietary fat in gliadin-immunologically sensitized mice, a morphological and statistical study of the intestinal mucosa was performed in two groups of animals.

One group of 3 animals was challenged with gluten and fed with a diet containing good quality olive oil and fish oil (GA); another group of 3 mice received a gluten enriched diet, containing sunflower oil (GB). Intestinal mucosal samples were taken after 7 days of receiving the challenge diet.

Animals challenged with gluten/olive and fish oil:

The mice of this group show intestinal mucosa with better preserved structure and higher digitiform villi compared to those who received the diet with sunflower oil (Fig. 18).

At higher magnification, it is possible to see the epithelium with irregular borders and a well-defined striated border of equal thickness throughout its length. The lamina propria lacks the inflammatory infiltrate observed in the animals challenged with the diet containing sunflower oil (Fig. 19).

Animals challenged with gluten/sunflower oil:

The intestines of these animals present conical villi, are shorter in height and have wider bases than the villi in the previously mentioned group. Increased inflammatory infiltrate in the lamina propria and increased mucosal thickness are observed. Large amount of cellular debris are observed in the intestinal lumen (Fig. 20 y 21).

One of the animals of this group presents a significant distortion of the ends of the villi and degenerative changes in the epithelial surface. At higher magnification, an intense inflammatory infiltrate of the lamina propria is confirmed. Vacuolar degeneration of the epithelial cells can be seen together with detachment of these cells and their remains appearing in the intestinal lumen (Fig. 22).

It is worth mentioning that the cell vacuolization is related to chronicity and irreversibility due to cell damage with epithelial degeneration and autolysis.

The alterations in the intestinal mucosa of this animal were evaluated at ultrastructural level. In the epithelium, it is possible to see areas with well-maintained absorptive cells which contrast with altered cells whose cytoplasms have lower electron density and vacuolization (Fig. 23a).

In the apical surface, it can be seen some areas with normal-appearing villi alternating with others with distorted microvilli, shorter in length, with widened globular ends (Fig. 23 b). Detached striated borders can also be seen in the intestinal lumen (Fig. 23 a).

The ends of several villi exhibit epithelial denudation. The cells that remain attached show the free surfaces of the lateral plasma membranes in the detachment zone. Numerous degenerating cell debris remain in the intestinal lumen (Fig. 23c).

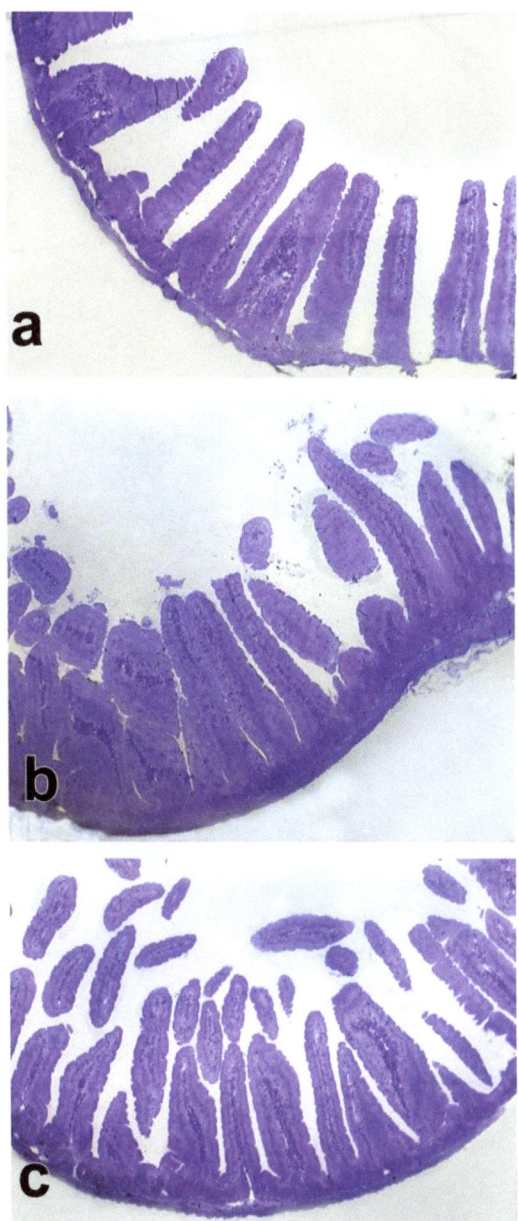

Figure 18 a, b and c: Microphotographs of intestinal mucosa from three animals sensitized with gliadin, challenged with gluten/good quality olive oil/fish oil. While some villi show a slight widening of the lamina propria, they maintain their digitiform structure. Araldite. TB.

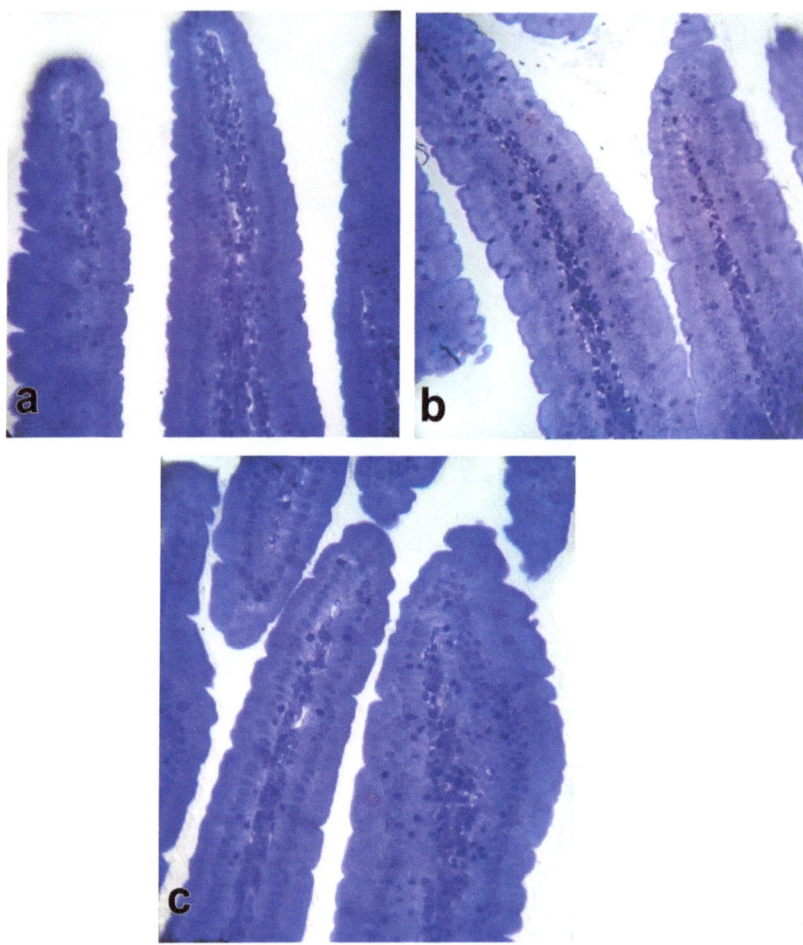

Figure 19 a, b and c. Microphotographs of intestinal villi from three animals of the group sensitized with gliadin, challenged with gluten/good quality olive oil/fish oil. The irregular edge of the epithelium and the presence of the striated border can be observed. The connective tissue axis have a normal appearance. Araldite. TB.

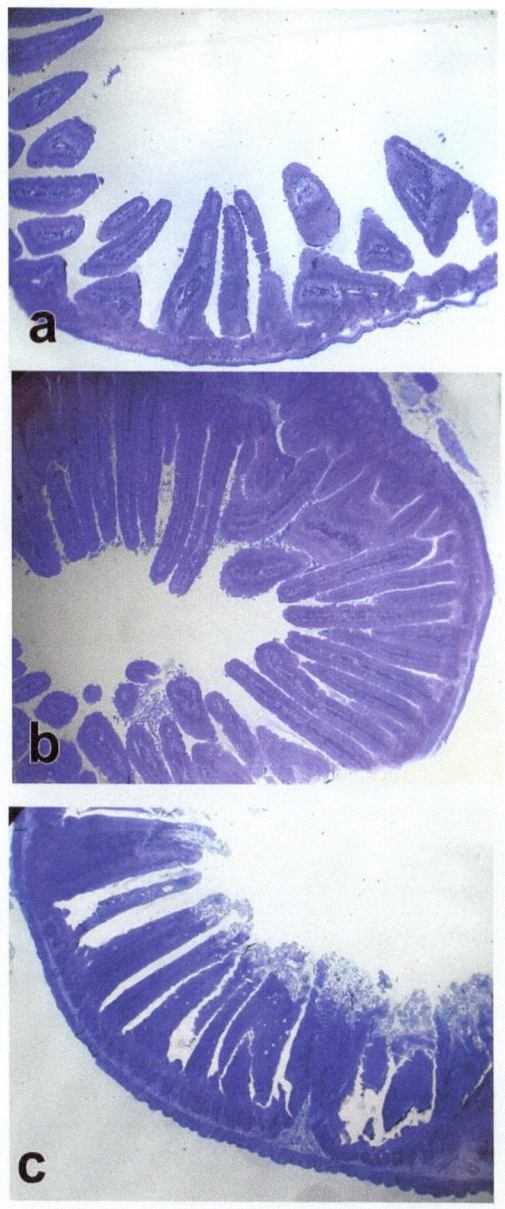

Figure 20 a, b and c. Microphotographs of intestine sections from three animals of the group sensitized with gliadin and challenged with gluten/sunflower oil. Villi with inflammatory infiltrate of the lamina propria causing widening of the mucosa can be seen. In one case (c), the ends of the villi distorted with degenerative changes in the epithelial surface are observed. Araldite. TB.

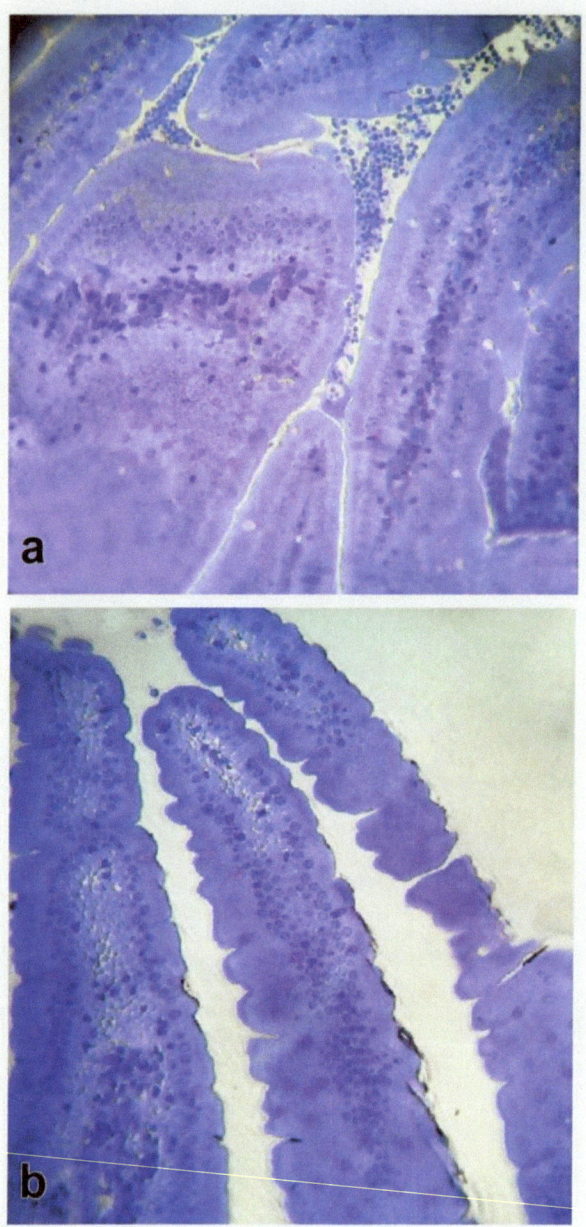

Figure 21 a and b. Microphotographs of longitudinal sections of intestinal villi from animals of the group sensitized with gliadin and challenged with gluten/sunflower oil. The infiltrate of the lamina propria and cellular debris in the lumen can be observed. Araldite. TB.

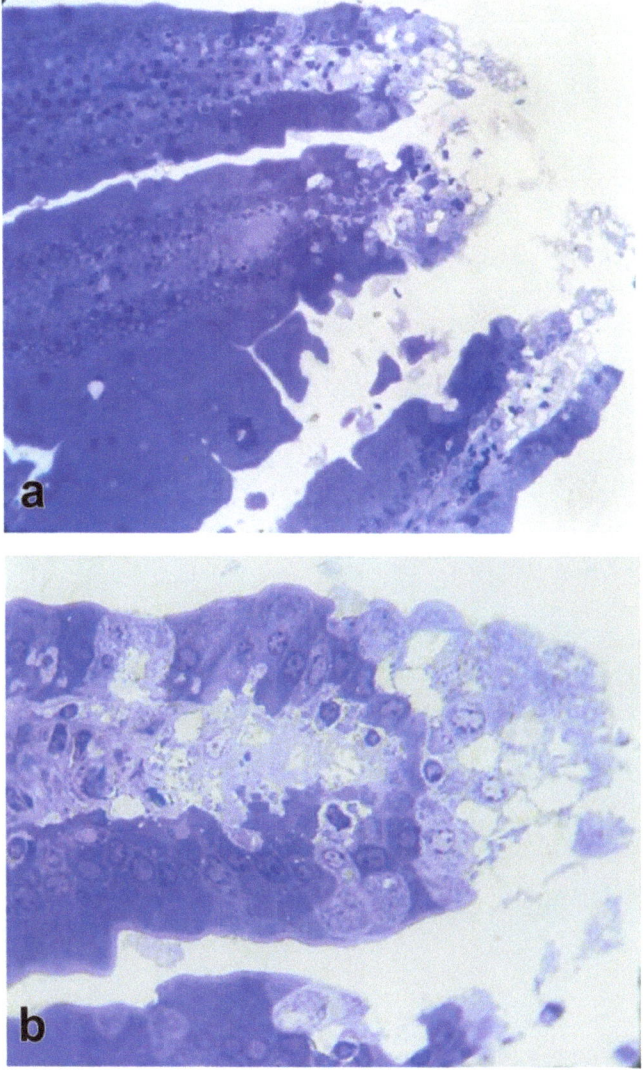

Figura 22 a and b. Microphotographs at higher magnification of an animal of the group challenged with gluten/sunflower oil. Degenerative processes are observed on the ends of the villi, with infiltrate of the lamina propria, vacuolation of the epithelial cells with detachment. Araldite. TB.

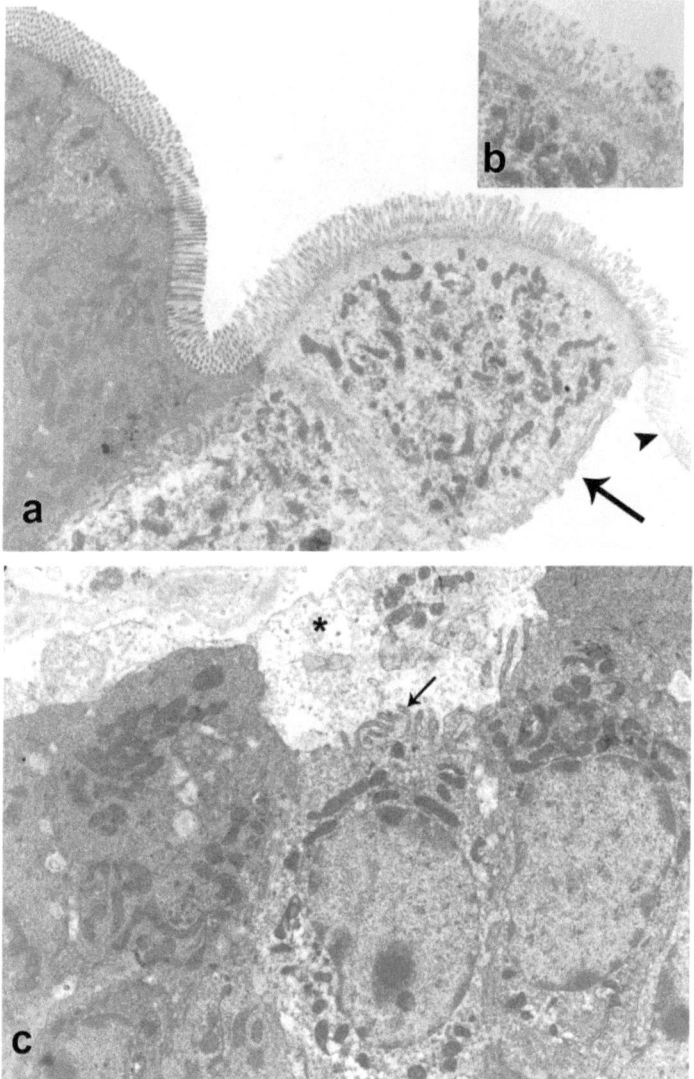

Figure 23. Electron micrographs of the intestinal epithelium of a mouse challenged with gluten/sunflower oil. a: Part of a cell with normal appearance (*) can be seen next two altered cells, with cytoplasms of lower electron density exhibiting a free lateral side (arrows), with detachment of the adjacent cell, where remains on the striated border (arrowhead) can be observed. Magnification: 3,600 Xb: Detail of distorted microvilli, with globular ends. Magnification: 10,000 X c: End of an intestinal villus showing epithelial cells with vacuoles and the detachment surface (arrows) of surface cells with debris remaining in the lumen (*). Magnification: 4,600 X

Statistical analysis:

In the animals of groups sensitized with gliadin and challenged with gluten and different types of fat, three parameters were statistically analyzed: height of villi, width of the bases and thickness of the intestinal mucosa: The recorded data are listed in Table 1.

Table 1. Effect of dietary fats in the morphology of the intestinal mucosa.

		Mean	SD
Height of villi	GA	3403.6	411.6*
	GB	2840.3	570.1
Width of the bases	GA	979.8	406.6
	GB	1184.5	4141
Thickness of the mucosa	GA	560.6	156.1*
	GB	821.3	258.6

GA: Mice immunized with gliadin and challenged with gluten/olive and fish oil (n = 3).

GB: Mice immunized with gliadin and challenged with gluten/sunflower oil (n = 3).
* $P < 0,001$ vs. GB

The animals that received a diet containing sunflower oil exhibit significantly shorter villi and a mucosa thicker than those fed with olive oil and fish (Fig. 24 and 26).

As regards the base width of the villi, although they are taller in animals challenged with sunflower oil, the difference was not statistically significant for this study variable (Fig. 25).

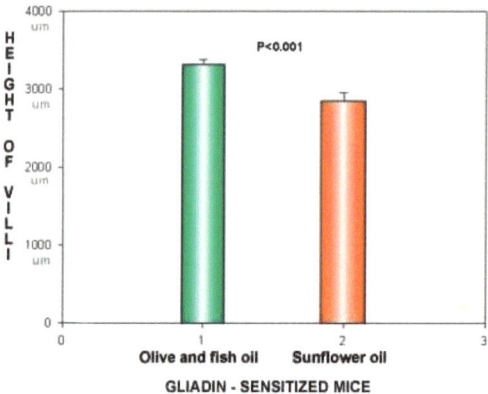

Figure 24: Height of villi in animals with different types of fat in the challenge diet (n = 6).

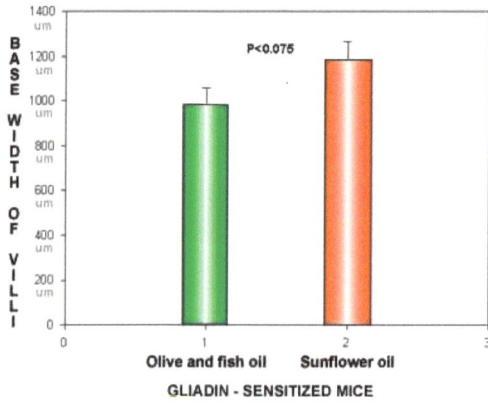

Figure 25: Base width of intestinal microvilli of animals challenged with gluten and different types of oil (n = 6).

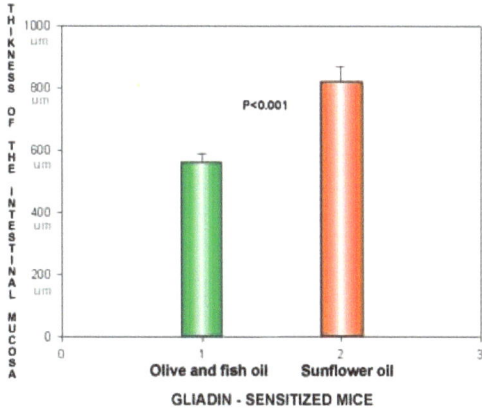

Figure 26: Thickness of the intestinal mucosa of mice challenged with a diet supplemented with different types of fat (n = 6).

Influence of cow's milk in the diet:

To study the effect of a diet with cow's milk in the morphology of the intestinal epithelium, three groups of gliadin-immunologically sensitized animals challenged with gluten incorporating or excluding the cow's milk for seven days were studied.

Animals challenged with gluten/sunflower oil/milk:

The intestinal mucosa of these animals exhibits has some conical villi, with widening of the lamina propria due to vascular dilation, hemorrhage, edema and inflammatory infiltrate.

In general, the tissue shows greater dye intensity (hyperchromasia). Prominent nuclei, separation between epithelial cells and surface cell detachment from the surface were observed (Fig. 27 y 28).

Animals challenged with gluten/low quality sunflower oil/milk:

The histological changes were exacerbated in animals that received a diet containing low quality olive oil and cow's milk, proving a greater degree of cell vacuolization and detachment of the surface cells of the epithelium in the ends of the villi.

It is worth highlighting the hyperchromasia in the sections and the greater space between the epithelial cells. In the lamina propria, significant areas of edema, vascular congestion and inflammatory infiltrate were observed (Fig. 29 and 30).

Animals challenged with gluten/low quality olive oil/exclusion of cow's milk:

In animals who do not receive cow's milk, the intestinal villi keep their digitiform shape, with more irregular borders. There is an increase in the number of goblet cells and the striated border is better preserved. In the lamina propria, less inflammatory infiltrate is seen and only few villi show a slight widening of the connective tissue central axis (Fig. 31). No hyperchromasia or cell vacuolization are observed, in contrast to the animals fed with diets containing cow's milk..

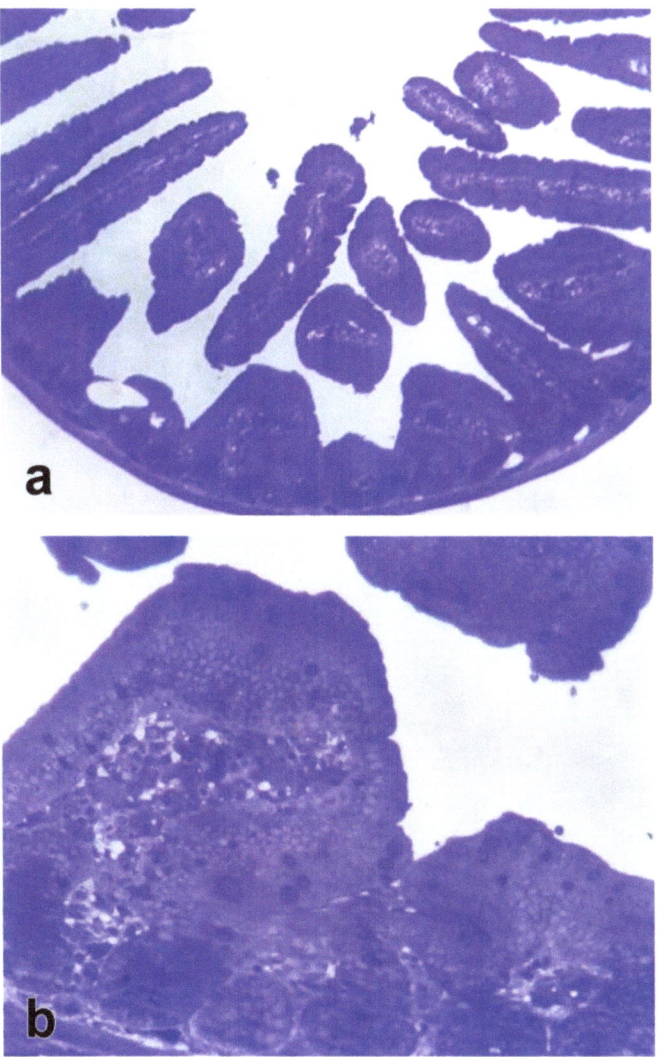

Figure 27. Microphotographs of intestinal mucosa of an animal sensitized to gliadin and challenged with gluten/sunflower oil/cow's milk. a: some villi exhibit widened bases. b: At higher magnification, it is possible to observe inflammatory cell infiltrate in the lamina propria and edema. Araldite. TB.

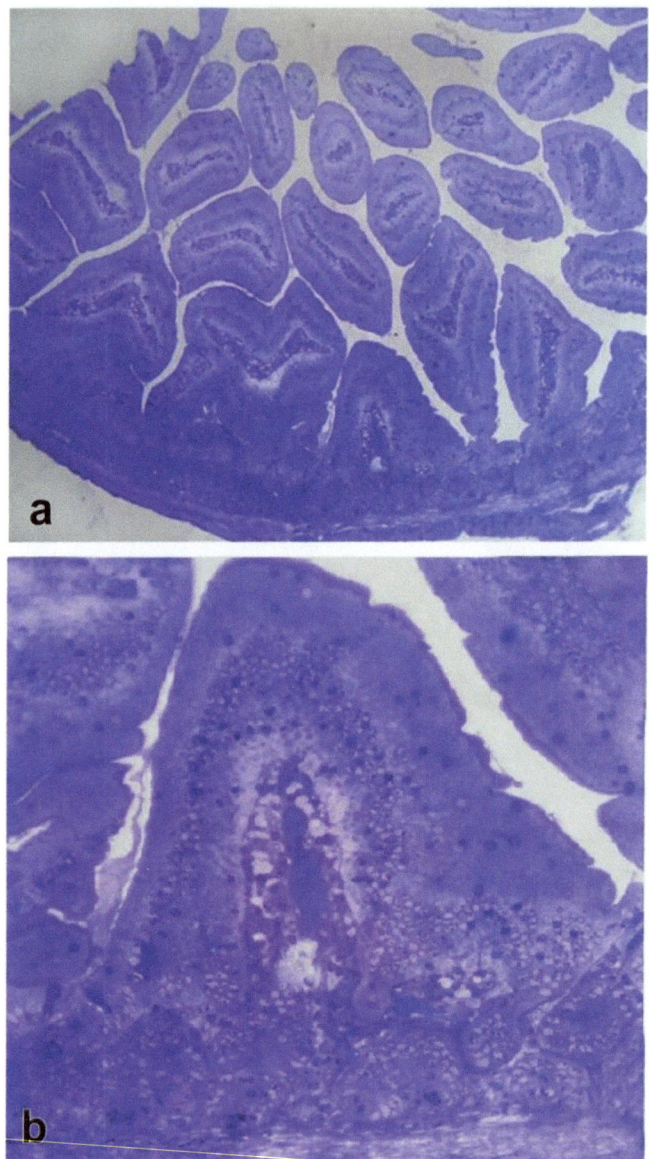

Figure 28. Cross section of the intestine of an animal immunized with gliadin and challenged with gluten/sunflower oil/cow's milk. a: The villi show architectural distortion with widening of the bases. b At higher magnification, it is possible to see inflammatory infiltrate in the lamina propria and edema with vascular changes: capillary congestion and hemorrhage. Araldite. TB.

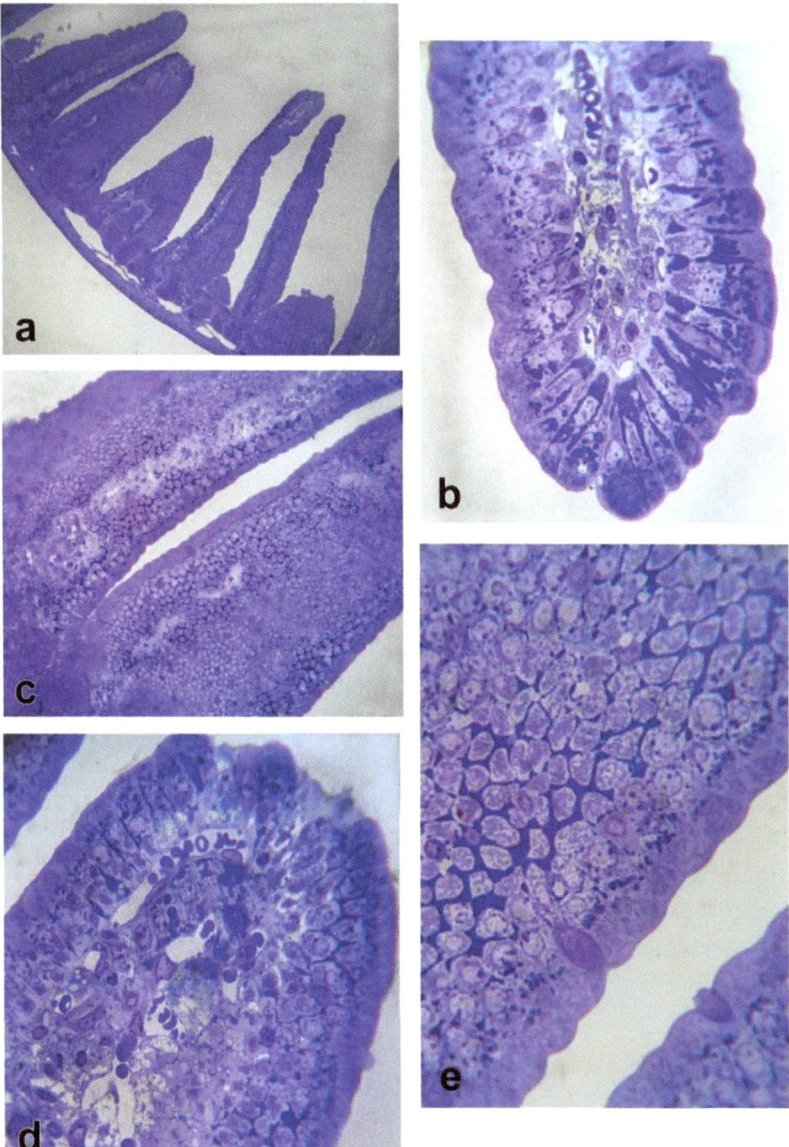

Figure 29 a-e: Microphotographs of intestine tissue sections from the group sensitized with gliadin and challenged with gluten/low quality olive oil/cow's milk. Cell hyperchromasia and intercellular spaces of the epithelium are observed. There is intense vascular congestion in the lamina propria and cytoplasmic vacuolization. Araldite. TB.

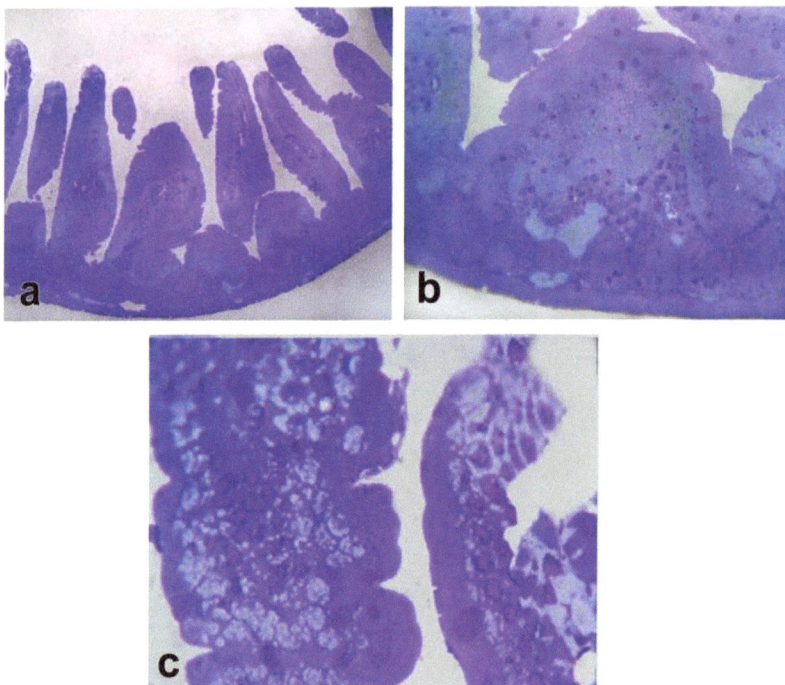

Figure 30. Microphotographs of intestinal mucosa from the group immunized with gliadin and challenged with gluten/low quality olive oil/cow's milk. a: Villi with widened bases are observed. b and c:At higher magnification, it can be seen edema, hemorrhage and marked cytoplasmic vacuolization of the epithelium in the lamina propria. Araldite. TB.

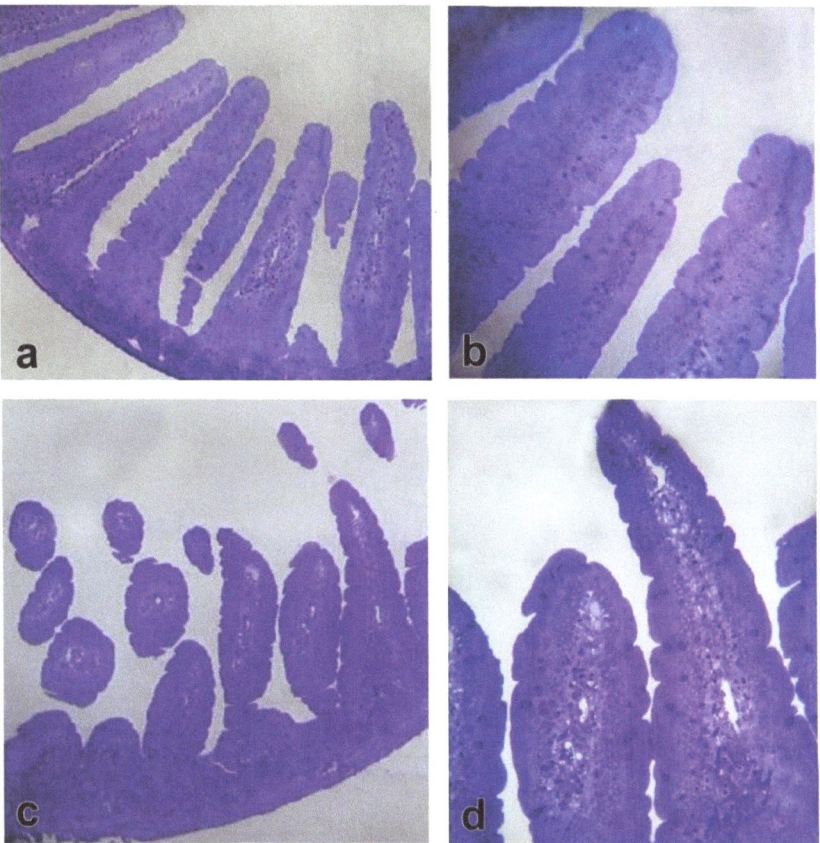

Figure 31 a-d. Microphotographs of intestinal mucosa sections from the group sensitized with gliadin and challenged with gluten/low quality olive oil/excluding cow's milk. The villi keep their height, digitiform appearance and irregular borders. Few villi show slight widening of the connective tissue central axis.

Electron microscopy:

For a better interpretation of the results of this stage of the research, the morphological characteristics of the intestinal mucosa of animals challenged with gluten incorporating or excluding cow's milk protein were studied at ultrastructural level.

In the intestinal mucosal of animals that received the diet incorporating cow's milk, large fat globules of low electron density are observed in the enterocytes, both in the apical, middle and basal area of the cytoplasm.

In some portions of the epithelium, these lipid globules occupy much of the cytoplasm, distorting the cell structure and limiting the organelles to small perinuclear and basal areas. Amongst the epithelial cells, more compact accumulations of lipid with higher electron density are seen (Fig. 32). In the apical surface, it is possible to see areas with alteration, shortening, deformity and separation of the microvilli.

In contrast with these conditions, the intestinal epithelial cells of immunologically sensitized animals that did not receive cow's milk in the diet exhibit lipid particles with characteristics and location different from the ones above mentioned. They are smaller, of similar diameter and higher electron density. They are not observed in the apical cytoplasm but near the nuclei of enterocytes (Fig. 33b). Thus, in cross sections that include different levels of epithelial cells, the lipid droplets appear in those including nuclei sections (Fig. 33a). Lipid accumulation are also seen between epithelial cells (intercellular spaces) in the basal area in the usual transit route of chylomicrons (Fig.33c). The apical microvilli generally preserve their uniform structure.

These observations at electron microscopy level highlight that the incorporation of cow's milk in the diet causes major alterations in the intestinal epithelium consisting mainly of storage of large globules of lipid substances in the cytoplasm, probably indicative of an altered transit.

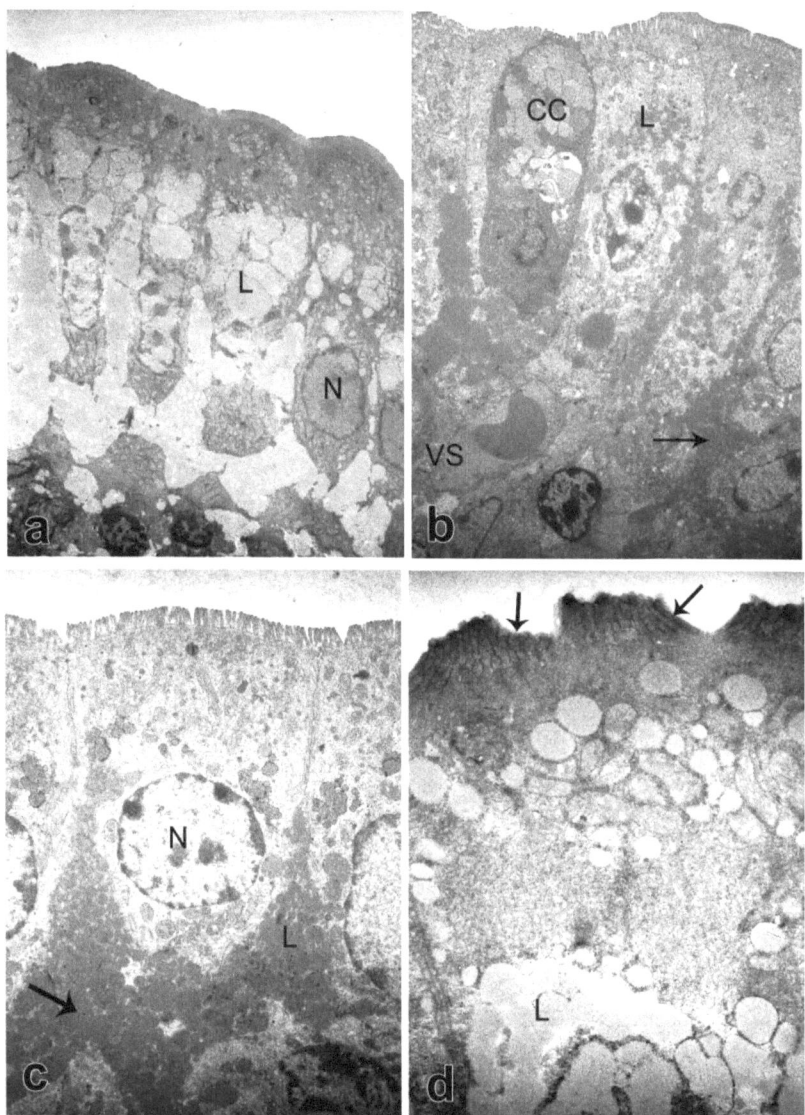

Figure 32 a-d: Electron microphotographs of the intestinal epithelium from a mouse sensitized with gliadin, challenged with gluten/low quality olive oil/cow's milk. Large globules of lipids (L) are observed in the cytoplasm. Lipid accumulations are also observed between the epithelial cells (arrows). In some areas, distortion of microvilli (arrowhead) is observed. GC: goblet cell. N: nuclei; a and b: magnification: 2,500 X, c: magnification: 4,200 X and d: magnification: 15,000 X.

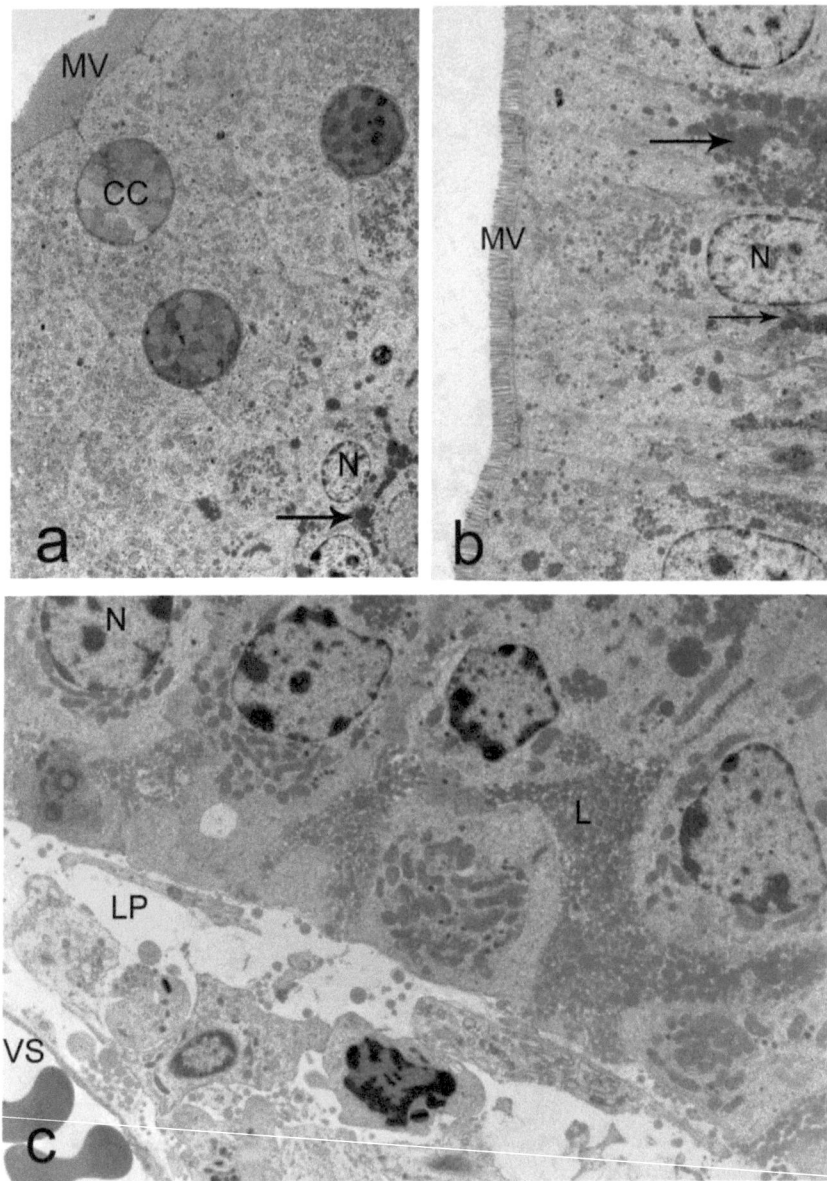

Figure 33: Electron microphotographs of the intestinal epithelium from a mouse immunized with gliadin, challenged with gluten/low quality olive oil/excluding cow's milk. a: cross-section and b longitudinal cut of the epithelium where high density small lipid droplets are observed in the perinuclear cytoplasm (arrows) at a magnification of 2,200 X. c: basal area of the epithelium with accumulation of lipid droplets (L) between the epithelial cells. Magnification: 2,800 X. GC: goblet cell. BV: blood vessel. LP: lamina propia.

Clinical cases:

There was clinical improvement in 80% of the patients studied after the completion of the diet prescribed despite wheat intake (disappearance of physical signs of the disease and good weight-height evolution). Eight patients became negative for anti-AG IgA and five became negative for anti-AG IgG. Four patients with positive results for AE before the diet, became negative for that antibody after the diet. In the remaining 20%, the positive antibodies and some symptomatic manifestations continued. In these cases, a biopsy of the proximal intestine confirmed the diagnosis of CD and a gluten-free diet was indicated. We show this series of 10 patients in the following table..

Case	Sex	Age	Weight	Height	Symptoms and Signs	Initial Lab Tests	Follow up
1	M	4 years and 6 months	23.0 kg	117 cm	Meteorism, irritability and afebrile seizures	Anti-AG IgG (+) Anti-AG IgA (+)	Anti-AG IgG (-) Anti-AG IgA (-) No meteorism, no repeated seizures, NWHE, normal brain CT scan
2	M	2 years and 3 months	12.8 kg	88 cm	Gingivitis, meteorism, recurrent abdominal pain	Anti-AG IgG (+) Anti-AG IgA (-) Anti-AE IgG (+) Anti-AE IgA (-)	Anti-AG IgG (-) Anti-AG IgA (+) Anti-AE IgG (-) Anti-AE IgA (-) Good general condition, NWHE
3	M	3 years and 8 months	14.5 kg	99 cm	Diarrhea and meteorism	Anti-AG IgG (+) Anti-AG IgA (+) AE IgG (-) AE IgA (-)	Anti-AG IgG (+) Anti-AG IgA (+) Anti-AE IgG (-) Anti-AE IgA (-) CD confirmed by biopsy
4	M	2 years and 11 months	14.6 kg	97 cm	meteorism, diarrhea, loss of appetite	Anti-AG IgG (+) Anti-AG IgA (+) Anti-AE IgG (-) Anti-AE IgA (-)	Anti-AG IgG (+) Anti-AG IgA (-) Anti-AE IgG (-) Anti-AE IgA (-) Normal abdomen, NWHE
5	M	4 years and 9 months	14.,5 kg	99 cm	diarrhea	Anti-AG IgG (+) Anti-AG IgA (+) Anti-AE IgG (-) Anti-AE IgA (-)	Anti-AG IgG (+) Anti-AG IgA (-) Anti-AE IgG (-) Anti-AE IgA (-) CD confirmed by biopsy
6	M	11 years and 10 months	40.0 kg	148 cm	Recurrent abdominal pain and meteorism	Anti-AG IgG (+) Anti-AG IgA (+)	Anti-AG IgG (+) Anti-AG IgA (-) No meteorism, NWHE
7	M	3 years and 3 months	18.4 kg	100 cm	meteorism, abdominal pain, cold and dermatitis	Anti-AG IgG (+) Anti-AG IgA (+) Anti-AE IgG (+) Anti-AE IgA (-)	Anti-AG IgG (-) Anti-AG IgA (-) Anti-AE IgG (-) Anti-AE IgA (-) Normal PE, NWHE
8	M	7 years and 1 month	24.9 kg	125 cm	meterorism, skin rash and eczema	Anti-AG IgG (+) Anti-AG IgA (+)	Anti-AG IgG (+) Anti-AG IgA (-) Normal abdomen without dermatitis, NWHE
9	F	4 years and 6 months	13.8 kg	100 cm	Meteorism, abdominal pain	Anti-AG IgA(+) Anti-AE IgA(+)	Anti-AG IgG(-) Anti-AE IgA(-) NWHE
10	M	4 years and 8 months	11.1 kg	96cms	diarrhea, vomit and meteorism	Anti-AG IgG (+) Anti-AG IgA (+) Anti-AE IgG (+) Anti-AE IgA (+)	AnAnti-AG IgG (-) Anti-AG IgA (-) Anti-AE IgG (-) Anti-AE IgA (-). NWHE

Table 2: Clinical and serological findings in the patients studied.

Abbreviations:
M: male; F: female; AG: anti-gliadin antibodies; AE: anti-endomysial autoantibodies,
PE: physical examination, NWHE: normal weight/ height evolution.

It is worth mentioning that when we analyzed fats and milk as variables, we contrasted again those variables in immunologically sensitized animals with the same method used in the group challenged with oats; however, the experience was repeated to compare differences amongst siblings, i.e., offspring of the same litter, this is why this latter groups were small in number.

DISCUSSION

Celiac disease (CD) is a disease related to alterations in the intestinal absorption, mediated by immunological factors in individuals genetically susceptible to foods containing wheat prolamins, oats, barley or rye, and that manifests itself through an inflammatory process of the small intestine mucosa.

CD has a high incidence and presents itself in different ways.

Lesions in the intestinal lining cause malabsorption syndrome and this in turn a state of malnutrition. The current and generally accepted treatment is lifelong exclusion of gluten from the diet of patients. At present there is no consensus about the potential toxicity of oats and its role in inducing CD.

Strict dietary compliance becomes very difficult due to the large number of commercial products containing these prolamins. This situation encouraged us to develop new experimental research that could provide data for a better understanding of the lesions and their interactions with other factors that may be critical in the expression and maintenance of the disease.

One of the most conspicuous limitations in the field of celiac disease research is the lack of a specific animal model, as noted by Shidrawi et al. (47).

The pathological changes in the intestinal mucosa are characteristic and manifest themselves with atrophy of the intestinal villi, inflammatory cell infiltrate and modification in the transport of nutrients and, in particular, lipids. Many of these lesions are superimposed with those that exhibit patients allergic to proteins in cow's milk. Cow's milk and gluten proteins, besides presenting common elements in their molecular structure, cause similar symptoms. In preparing food, proteins have a characteristic high viscosity which can vary with the modification of the type of fat. In this way, it could be possible to relate these three elements commonly consumed: wheat, milk and fat.

In bread making, insoluble proteins containing gliadin and glutein are hydrated, and wheat flour becomes a viscoelastic dough able to retain the gases generated during the fermentation process. With the addition of water, insoluble proteins form a three-dimensional lattice with hydrogen and disulfide bridges. Disulfide bridges play a major role in the formation of gluten.

The viscosity of the intestinal content reduces the digestibility of nitrogen, starch, lipids and amino-acids present in the lumen (4) because it creates a protective layer in the chyme against the action of digestive enzymes (48).

At an acid pH, the casein in milk becomes completely insoluble due to the formation of a web of flocs that affect the penetration. Thus, physicochemical characteristics such as adhesiveness, viscosity and capacity of penetration influencing the processes of digestion and absorption of nutrients are combined.

The development of an accessible experimental model, as the one presented in this thesis, allowed the analysis of these variables and the study the changes occurring in the intestine of sensitized animals when foods such as cereals, milk and fats are combined.

In our experimental model, we used BALB male and female mice whose mothers were subjected to a special gluten-free diet; this diet was also used for the offspring after weaning. These mice were immunologically sensitized from the sixth week of weaning, by injecting purified antigen (gliadin or avenin) emulsified with Freund's adjuvant. A booster injection was repeated two weeks later. The immunoreactivity to these proteins was assessed on the fifteenth day after the second injection with the addition of the "problematic" protein to the diets. These challenge diets varied based on the experimental protocol; to this end, gluten-free base diets were enriched with gluten or oats, modifying the fat composition with the addition of extra virgin olive oil of different qualities. Finally the variable of incorporating or excluding cow's milk in the diet was also evaluated.

The epithelium of the intestinal mucosa of normal mice and control animals immunized with gliadin and avenin do not differ in their structural organization and exhibit a strong resemblance to the human intestinal epithelium obtained from normal patients. The intestinal villi have a digitiform, regular morphology and are lined by simple columnar epithelium made up of polarized cells. Its most distinctive element is a regular cover of microvilli and the glycocalyx on its apical pole clearly individualized in microphotographs observed under an electron microscope. At photon microscopy level, this structure has the typical brush border morphology.

The challenge with gluten and oats in these sensitized animals causes characteristic changes in the intestinal epithelium. The villi lose their typical histologic conformation and become more irregular, with widened bases, acquiring a pyramidal shape. In addition, an inflammatory cell infiltrate is detected in the lamina propria. Observing these lesions under the electron microscope reveals degenerative changes in the epithelial cells and distortion of the villi with vacuolization and lipid globules accumulation in the cytoplasm. Often compact accumulations of lipids are also seen in the intercellular spaces.

These results allow us to confirm that with our protocols it is possible to achieve an adequate sensitization and a well-defined immune reactivity to gliadin and avenin in mice, in contrast to what Troncone and Ferguson (58) described. They stated that the injection of purified gliadin in itself was not a sufficient condition for positive immune reactivity. For a proper immune reactivity in mice, these authors performed a series of experimental studies that introduced factors as variable as the induction of anaphylaxis by infection with *Nippopastrongylus brasiliensis* larvae and the induction of graft versus host reaction through the intraperitoneal injection of splenic cells.

In our study, the first parenteral sensitization tests were performed with incomplete Freund's adjuvant, but then sensitization was enhanced combining a first injection of complete adjuvant followed by a second injection with incomplete adjuvant. Adjuvants allow the slow release of the antigen and a persistent antigenic stimulation is achieved.

Having achieved a reliable experimental model, the next step in our work was to evaluate the potential toxicity of oats in celiac disease.
In recent years, specialists of different countries (14, 6, 57, 22, 50, 20) have introduced the intake of oats in celiac patients and patients with dermatitis herpetiformis, taking into account that various studies have shown that a

moderate amount of oats could be a safe food for them. According to experiments carried out in vivo and in vitro with different age groups exposed to different amounts of oats, with a variable duration of exposure to the challenges, it was concluded that oats is an acceptable food for celiac patients, whose diet is marked by serious constraints. However, although this issue has been extensively discussed, it has not been sufficiently analyzed, and other work groups that show the harmful effects of oats in celiac patients have emerged. In relation to this issue, there are numerous publications that expose serious contradictions as regards the intake of oats. Janatuinen et al. (22, 23) described that challenges with small amounts of oats did not cause changes in the architecture of the villi in adult celiac patients.

According to a study published by Srinivasan et al. (50) ten adult patients with celiac disease in clinical remission and histological normalization were given 50 g of oats daily for 12 weeks while maintaining a strict gluten-free diet. The cereal was analyzed to discard possible contamination with gluten. Clinical trials and dosages of anti-gliadin and anti-endomysium antibodies were serially performed at baseline, 1, 4 and 12 weeks.

Endoscopic biopsies were taken before the administration of oats and at end of the study and no morphological alterations of the intestinal villi or changes in clinical and laboratory parameters were detected.

In contrast with these results, we can mention Arentz-Hansen et al. (5) who studied 9 adult patients with celiac disease who received a daily amount of 50 g of oats with their diet. Four of these patients had clinical symptoms of celiac disease and three of them had inflammation typical of the disease after exposure to oats. Leone et al. (26) also found alterations in the intestinal mucosa; they also observed in intestinal biopsy specimens that oat prolamins may cause an immune reaction.

The contribution we make to this discussion with our experimental model is that histopathological changes of the intestinal mucosa were detected both in mice challenged with wheat and in mice challenged with oats. The parenteral administration of avenin followed by challenge diets caused a disruption of the villous structure with the same dose used for the gliadin sensitization. The response we achieved by incorporating the immunogenic proteins was comparable in the group receiving a gluten enriched diet and in the group receiving the oats enriched diet. The immunogen administration protocol used to achieve the sensitization of these proteins in mice was similar to the doses and routes of administration described by Troncone and Ferguson (58).

In this research, in addition to the great similarity in the intestinal reactivity with challenge diets with gliadin and avenin, we also proved a cross-reactivity between the two proteins, which allow us to understand the role of oats in the pathogenesis of celiac disease and interpret the discrepancies in the discussions generated by this immune mechanism.

Cross-reactivity between prolamines has also been the subject of several controversies. The observations recorded for celiac disease exhibit a certain similarity with the behavior detected in patients with allergy to grass pollen, which also shows a blatant cross-reactivity with different pollens. Hardman et al. (20) studied ten adult patients (seven men and three women) with a mean age of 58 years suffering from dermatitis herpetiformis, microscopically confirmed in skin biopsies. These patients followed a strict gluten-free diet and then oats which had been rigorously controlled to confirm it was free from contamination was added. Under these conditions and for a period of 12 weeks, no adverse effects of oats were detected in serological tests (anti-gliadin antibodies, antireticulin antibodies and anti-endomysium antibodies), intestine and skin biopsies. Parnell, Ellis and Ciclitira (37) in a letter to the editor about the Hardman et al. article suggested that moderate amounts of oats can be included in the diet of celiac patients. However, they consider unwise to advise gluten sensitive patients that oats can be safely consumed. They also express that the absence of toxicity of oats has not yet been clearly proven. In a reply to these authors, Hardman and Fry (20) describe the possibility of developing monoclonal antibodies against such small epitopes with only 6 amino-acid residues and state that the antibodies against fragments of 19 amino-acids may not be specific to celiac disease since the epitope best known to be active is the 12 amino-acids epitope. A similar result was described by Ellis et al. (15) but using as immunogenic material a gliadin fragment with a larger sequence (19 amino-acids), which exhibits a stronger reactivity to oats peptides.

Hardman and Fry (20) report that although the size of the epitopes would be related to the cross-reactivity between gliadin and avenin, the monoclonal antibodies against wheat enteropathic peptides do not prove the toxicity of oats. They further argue that peptides of different nature can be absorbed by celiac patients and induce the production of antibodies, although they also explain that so far, there is no evidence that these antibodies may have a primary pathogenic role.

As a clinical observation, the effects of oats on the symptoms of celiac patients were initially described by Dicke et al. (12) in celiac children were steatorrhea manifested by the incorporation of oats into the diet was observed. Subsequently, Baker et al. (6) verified alterations in the D-xylose incorporating oats during the follow-up of 12 adult and pediatric patients with celiac disease. On the other hand, Picarelli et al. (41) reported that in cultures of duodenal mucosa biopsy specimens of celiac patients in clinical remission, anti-endomysial antibodies were not detected by indirect immunofluorescence in the supernatant of these cultures after incubation for 72 h in media containing high concentrations of avenin (2 g/L).

Research published by Lundin et al., University of Oslo, with the participation of the Gluten Unit of the National Center for Biotechnology (CSIC) of Spain, under the supervision of Enrique Mendez, confirmed for the first time the development of symptoms of malabsorption and impairment of the intestinal mucosa in a celiac patient caused by the consumption of oats (27). For this research, 19 adult celiac patients were enrolled. They received 50 grams of oats daily for 12 weeks. The Spanish team analyzed the components of the different types of oats available and selected one free from wheat, barley or rye contamination. One of the celiac patients was sensitive to oats and the intestinal biopsy showed that oats caused a partial atrophy of the intestinal mucosa, which was solved with the exclusion of oats from the diet; however, the patient had a relapse with subtotal atrophy of the intestinal villi and acute dermatitis when oats was incorporated into their diet again.

As a new contribution, after the completion of this thesis, it was determined that both gliadin and avenin are potentially toxic to celiac patients. During the handling of these proteins, we found that gliadin has more viscosity and adhesiveness which, in everyday life, can mean that more quantities of oats (in comparison to wheat) are needed to produce lesions in sensitized individuals. In a second stage of this research, a possible interaction of lipids in celiac disease was studied. For this purpose, we examined changes in the intestinal morphometry caused by the type and quality of fats incorporated into the challenge diets of gliadin-sensitized mice. In recent years, numerous and different investigations have been published on dietary lipids to assess the role they might have on certain intestinal diseases. For example, Bellido et al. (7) observed in eight normolipidemic volunteers that cytotoxicity, measured as LDH activity and induced by triglyceride-rich lipoproteins determined after the intake of a meal containing butter, was superior to that produced by a meal rich in virgin olive oil and nuts. Hennig et al. (21) studied the disruption of the endothelial barrier by lipolytic remnants of a diet rich in lipoproteins. Rocío Abia et al. (1) noted that chylomicrons formed after following the diet including sunflower oil remained longer in blood than those generated by the diet with virgin olive oil.

In the presence of lipid molecules, the water forces the hydrophobic molecules into a cage-shaped structure that reduces the mobility of lipids. The hydrophobic tails tend to interact with each other, creating a hydrophobic space from which water is expelled, and in which other hydrophobic molecules can also be trapped, while the polar head interacts with water (42).

In the presence of water, the hydrophobic effect makes amphipathic lipids expose the important property of their self-structuring leading to three different types of structures: micelles (monolayers) and vesicles (or bilayers).

In inflammatory conditions, edema of the intestinal villi due to the accumulation of interstitial fluid is observed; this situation can cause alterations in the absorption and transit of lipids in the intestinal epithelium, which can interact directly with the structural tissue damage.

Encouraged by these investigations, we decided to study the absorption of lipids in the intestine in gliadin-immunologically sensitized animals challenged with gluten.

Our results showed a strong correlation between the disruption of villous architecture and the type of fat added to the diet. The alterations of intestinal villi we observed were more notorious when sunflower oil was used; also, the protection of the intestinal morphology was confirmed when the main source of dietary fat was good quality olive oil and fish oil. Lavado et al. (25) reported that oleic acid inhibits the permeability of intercellular junctions in rat astrocytes in primary culture.

Regarding the research we carry out in this area, it is worth mentioning that the oleic acid present in certain vegetable oils, such as olive oil, avocado oil and, to a lesser extent, grape seed oil, is a monounsaturated fatty acid having a double bond near the center of the hydrocarbon chain, a characteristic that creates a twist in the molecule.

Some fatty acids having more than one double bond are individualized as polyunsaturated fatty acids, i.e., they have multiple twists. These twists prevent molecules (42) from packaging tightly. This characteristic suggests that lipids rich in polyunsaturated fatty acids, like sunflower oil, would follow a different transit route in the enterocyte.

With the use of challenge diets rich in gluten and sunflower oil in mice immunologically sensitized to gliadin, we could confirm intestinal lesions characterized by edema, vascular congestion and inflammatory infiltrate, in addition to accumulations of fat globules in the cytoplasm of epithelial cells and in the intercellular spaces extending to areas near the apical surface of the epithelium. This feature enables us to speculate that the edema initially limited to the lamina propria of the mucosa can reach shallower areas of the intestinal epithelium causing an obstacle in the transit of lipids, which in turn contributes to greater disruption of the intestinal villi architecture.

The discovery of large fat globules in epithelium biopsies of patients with celiac disease and allergies to the proteins of cow's milk was described by Variend et al. (60). Smaller globules in the deeper areas of the lamina propria have been linked to postenteritis syndrome and lactase deficiency.

In gliadin-immunologically sensitized mice challenged with gluten, a decline in the number and size of the lipid inclusions in the intestinal mucosa was detected when cow's milk was excluded from the diet and sunflower oil was replaced with olive oil.

In this last stage of the research on celiac disease, the information obtained experimentally was used in the personal clinical practice.

Patients with positive results for high specificity antibodies for celiac disease, such as anti-gliadin IgA antibodies, anti-endomysial antibodies and, in some cases, anti-tissue transglutaminase, with clinical signs such as meteorism, weight/height deceleration, afebrile seizures, recurrent respiratory infection, diarrhea and constipation, were subjected to a complete diet with gluten; however, cow's milk was excluded and the consumption of beef was reduced. This protocol allowed the reversion of symptoms of the disease and, in some patients, an unexpected observation of negative results for anti-gliadin and anti-endomysial antibodies in the blood despite the fact that the patients continued with wheat consumption. This diet was maintained, on average, for an initial period of two months before deciding to obtain biopsies to diagnose the celiac disease and indicate a permanent gluten-free diet. In many of these patients, the intestinal biopsy has not been performed because the patients are in good health conditions and present negative antibodies, while following a diet without beef protein (or in very low quantities) with calcium supplements and vitamin D.

It is possible that these results may be considered evidence of peptide pathogenicity of a different nature than that in wheat, as it is the case in cow's milk.

Our observations support the conclusion that intolerance to cow's milk would not only be a trigger of celiac disease or a consequence of it, but also one of the main factors causing the disease in genetically predisposed individuals, which has a strong implication in the current diagnostic protocol.

After completing this research and performing an analysis of the results, it is worth noting that not only wheat and oats have an important role in the pathogenesis of celiac disease, but other molecules such as proteins from cow's milk and lipids, may be playing a leading role in this disease. This suggests that in case we see a patient with signs and symptoms of celiac disease, it may be wise to take a reasonable time for observation, exclude derivative of cow's milk and beef proteins, recommend the use of good quality oils, clinically reexamine the patient and order laboratory tests. If any alteration persists despite these measures, an intestinal biopsy must be requested. Thus, the results will be more accurate and could provide better basis for the diet to be followed.

The experimental findings already applied in the clinical practice are allowing to reverse the immunological and clinical alterations in some patients who once would have been labeled as celiac, without excluding the wheat from the diet. This lays the foundations of a new and interesting debate on food allergy and provides a suitable experimental model for new contributions on this subject.

Personally, I consider very valuable the findings that contribute to expand the current understanding of an autoimmune disease that is treated with changes in eating habits.

CONCLUSION

The sensitization protocols to gliadin and avenin through parenteral immunization followed by challenge diets were effective in achieving a well-standardized experimental model with laboratory animals that can be reproduced in new research related to intestinal absorption and food allergy.

Histopathological alterations were observed not only in challenges with gluten but also in challenges with oats, and these changes were more evident when the challenge diet was performed with the protein opposite to that used for the immunization. In this way, the role of oats in the pathogenicity of celiac disease is confirmed, making an important contribution to the current discussion worldwide on this subject.

The modification of the oils used in the challenge diet caused varying degrees of intestinal lesions; the lesions with the highest severity were those caused by the diet containing sunflower oil or low quality olive oil, compared to good quality olive oil combined with fish oil. This finding was used in the clinical practice to advise patients in the process of gluten sensitization against consuming low quality oils especially together with foods with wheat flour; avoiding these foods helped reverse intolerance.

The exclusion of cow's milk from the challenge diet with gluten in gliadin-sensitized animals caused less severe lesions of the intestinal villi. This allows to suggest the participation of cow's milk in the pathogenesis of CD.

The results obtained in this research on celiac disease show histological evidence that molecules other than cereal prolamines, such as vegetable oil fats and proteins from cow's milk, may accompany wheat in the genesis of this pathology.

APPENDIX:
A story to share

One day, something happened to me that sums up my desire to share this book with you. While in my office, I ordered an intestinal biopsy for a patient since, despite clinical improvement, he was still positive for anti-wheat antibodies after following a diet excluding milk and incorporating good quality oils. The patient did not return for a long time. Almost a year later, this teenager came to see me and said, - "Dr., I had lost my health insurance coverage, that's the reason I couldn't return. But now, I have coverage again that this why I've come back". I was quite worried and I said, "You tested positive even for the most specific antibodies." - "Why did not you come to find a solution?" And he said, - "Dr., don't worry, I'm fine". - "What diet are you using?", I asked. And he replied - "I eat gluten, but I don't drink milk, I'm very careful with the oils I use and use the calcium and the vitamin you prescribed me". - "Right", I said. "But you have to do the preoperative analysis and do the antibodies lab tests again", I said while thinking about asking for an endoscopy.

To my surprise, the patient who looked good, felt good and was growing well tested negative for all the antibodies while consuming gluten. Why would I then request a biopsy? I kept monitoring him. He's doing very well and if he hadn't lost his health insurance coverage, he would have undergone the biopsy when all his antibodies tested positive. Surely, I would have found lesions and would have indicated a lifelong gluten-free diet.

Many questions... many doors that open to debate... a complex issue, but there is light at the end of the tunnel.

BIBLIOGRAFÍA

1-Abia R., Perona J., Pacheco Y., Montero E., Muriano F., Ruiz Gutierrez V. 1999. Postprandial triacilglycerols from dietary virgin olive oil are selectively cleared in humans. J Nutr 129:2184-2191.

2-Ammerman AJ., Cavalli-Sforza LL. 1971. Measuring the rate of spread of early farming in Europe Man 6:674-671.

3-Annison G. 1991. Relationship between the levels of solublenonstarch polysaccharides and the apparent metabolizable energy of wheats assayed in broiles chikens. J Agric Food Chem 39:1252-1256.

4-Arentz-Hansen H., Fleckenstein B., Molberg O., Scott H., Koning F., Jung G., Roepstorff P., Lundin KEA., Sollid M. 2004. The Molecular Basis for Oat Intolerance in Patients with Celiac Disease .PLoS Med. 1:84-92.

5-Astruc J. 1760. Diarrhea of infants. Capítulo XVIII. Traité des maladies des Femmes. París. Segunda Edición.

6-Baker PG., Read AE. 1976. Oats and barley toxicity in celiac patients. Postgrad Med J 52:264-8.

7-Bellido C., López M., Blanco J-Colio LM., Pérez-Martínez P., Suriana FJ., Martín –Ventura JL. 2004. Butter and walnuts, but not olive oil, elicit postprandial activation of nuclear transcription factor kappa B in peripheral blood mononuclear cells from healthy male volunteers .Am J Clin Nutr 80:1487-91.

8-Cappadocia A. 100. Corpus Medicorum Graecorum II. Hude C. Segunda Edición. Academia de Ciencias de Berlín .

9-Charbonier L., Jos J., Mougenot JF., Mosse J. 1980. Comparative toxicity of different cereals for subjects intolerant of gluten. Reprod Nutr Dev 20:1369-77.

10-Chorzelski TP., Beutner EH., Sulej J., Tchorzewska H., Jablonska H., Kumar V., Kapuscinska A. 1984. IgA anti-endomysium antibody. A new immunological marker of dermatitis herpetiformis and celiac disease. Br J Dermatol 111:395-402.

11-De Robertis E., Hib J. 2004. Fundamentos de Biología celular y molecular de De Robertis. Editorial El Ateneo. Cuarta Edición. Bs As. Argentina.

12-Dicke WK., Weigers HA., Van de Kamer JH.. 1953.The presence in wheat of a factor having a deleterious effect in cases of celiac disease .Coeliac DiseaseII. Acta Paediatr Scandinavica (Uppsala) 42:34-42.

13-Dietrich W., Ehnis T., Bauer M. 1997. Identification of tissue transglutaminase as the autoantigen of coeliac disease. Nature Med 3:797-801.

14-Dissanayake AS., Truelove SC., Whitehead R. 1974. Lack of harmful effect of oats on small-intestinal mucosa in celiac disease. Br Med J 4:189-91.

15-Ellis HJ., Freedman AR., Ciclitira PJ. 1989.The production and characterisation of monoclonal antibodies to wheat gliadin peptides. J Immunol Methods 120:17-22.

16-Fennema OR. 1985. Introducción a la Ciencia de los Alimentos. Editorial Reverté. Barcelona.

17-Gartner LP., Hiatt JL. 1997. Histología texto y atlas Editorial Mc Graw-Hill Interamericana traducido de la primera edición en inglés. México.

18-Gee SJ. 1888. On the Coeliac affection. St Bartolomew´s Hosp Rep 24:17-20.

19-Hadjivassiliou M., Gibson A., Davies- Jones GA., Lobo AJ., Stephenson TJ., Milford –Ward A. 1996. Does cryptic gluten sensitivity play a part in neurological illness? Lancet 347:369-371.

20-Hardman CM., Garioch JJ., Leonard JN. ,Thomas HJW., Walker M., Path FRC., Lortan JE., Lister A., Fry L., MD. 1997. Absence of toxicity of oats in patients with dermatitis herpetiformis. N Engl J Med 337:1884-1887.

21-Hennig B., Chung BH., Watkins BA. 1992. Disruption of endothelial barrier function by lipolytic remmants of trigliceride-rich lipoproteins. Atherosclerosis 95:235-247.

22-Janatuinen EK., Pikkaraines PH., Kemppainen TA., KosmoV-M., Jarvinem RMK., Matti IJ., Julkunen RJK. 1995. A comparison of diets with and without oats in adults with celiac disease. N Engl J Med 333:1033-1037.

23-Janatuinen EK., Kemppoinen TA. 2000. Lack of cellular and humoral immunological responses to oats in adults with coeliac disease. Gut 46:327-31.

24-Köhler P., Belitz H-D., Wieser H. 1993. Disulphide bonds in wheat gluten: further cystine peptides from high molecular weight and low molecular weight subunits of glutenin and from γ-gliadins. Z Lebensm Unters Forsch 196:239-247.

25-Lavado E., Sánchez-Abarca LI., Tabernero A., Bolaños JP., Medina JM. 1996. Efecto del ácido oleico sobre la comunicación intercelular en astrocitos de rata durante el desarrollo. *Ars Pharmaceutica* 37:739-751 .

26-Leone NA., Mazzarella G., Ciacci C., y col. 1996. Oats prolamines in Vitro activate intestinal cell-mediated immunity in coeliac disease. In: Collin P., Maki M., eds. All on Coeliac Disease. Free Paper Abstracts Seventh International Symposium on Coeliac Disease September 5-7 Tampere, Finland.

27-Lundin KEA., Nilsen EM., Scott HG., Loberg EM., Gjoen A., Brotlie J., Mendez SkarVE., Lovik A., Kett K. 2003. Oats induced villous atrophy in celiac disease. Gut 52:1649-1652.

28-Mackey J., Treem WR., Worley G., Money A Hart P Kishnani PS. 2001. Frequency of celiac disease in individuals with Down syndrome in the United States. Clin Pediatr (Phila). 40:249-252.

29-Maiuri L., Ciacci C., Auricchio S., Brown V., Quaratino S., Londei M. 2000. Interleukin 15 mediates epithelial changes in celiac disease. Gastroenterology 119:996-1006.

30-McDonald WC., Dobbins WO III., Rubin CE..1965. Studies of the familial nature of celiac sprue using biopsy of the small intestine. N Engl J Med 272:448-456.

31-Maluenda C., Phllips AD., Briddon A., Walker-Smith JA. 1984. Quantitative analysis of small intestinal mucosa in cow´s milk sensitive enteropathy. J Pediatr Gastroenterol Nutr 3:349-356.

32-Manuel García M. 2003. La enfermedad celíaca hoy. Vox Paediatrica 1:37-42.

33-Marsh MN. 1992. Gluten, major histocompatibility complex, and the small intestine. A molecular and immunobiologic approach to the spectrum of gluten sensivity ("celiac sprue"). Gastroenterology 102:330-54.

34-Maurano F., Siciliano RA D., De Giulio B., Luongo D., Mazzeo MF., Troncone R., Auricchio S., Rossi M. 2001. Intranasal administration of one alpha gliadin can down regulate the Immune reponse to a whole gliadin in mice. Scand J Immunol 53:290-295.

35-Meeuwisse GW. 1970. Diagnostic criteria in celiac disease. Acta Paediatr Scand 59:461-465.

36-Melter M., Belitz H-D., Gellerman B., Wieser H., Stern M. 1988. Hadling of gliadin peptides B1-B4 and of cow's milk proteins by rat jejunum gut sacs. J Pediatr Gastroenterol Nutr 7:196-202.

37-Parnell N., Ellis HJ. Ciclitira P. 1998. Absence of toxicity of oats in patients with dermatitis herpetiformis. Correspondence. N England J Med 338:1470-1471.

38-Paulley JW. 1954. Observations on the aetiology of idiopathic steatorrhoea. Br Med J 2:1318-1321.

39-Perez-Moreno M., Jamora C. 2003. Fuchs E. Sticky business: orchestrating cellular signals at adherens junctions. Cell. 112:535-548.

40-Phillips AD., Rice SJ., France NE., Walker-Smith JA. 1979. Small intestinal intraepithelial lymphocyte levels in cow's milk protein intolerance. Gut 20:509-12.

41-Picarelli A., Di Tola M., Sabbatella L., Gabrielli F., Di Cello T., Anania MC., Mastracchio A., Silano M., De Vincenzi M. 2001. Immunologic evidence of no harmful effect of oats in celiac disease. Am J Clin Nutr 74:137-40.

42-Porter HP., Saunders DR., Tytget G., Brunser O., Rubin CE. 1971. Fat absortion in bile fistula man. A morphological and biochemical study. Gastroenterology 60:1008-1019.

43-Purves W., Sadava D., Orians G., Heller HC. 2003. Vida Sexta Edición. La Ciencia de la Biología. Editorial Médica Panamericana. España. Cap.3, Macromoléculas su química y biología p49-50.

44-Reunala T., Collin P. 1997. Diseases associated with dermatitis herpetiformis. Br J Dermatol 136:315-318.

45-Ribes-Konickx C., Gilian JP., Polanco I., Peña AS. 1984. IgA Antigliadin Antibodies in Cloeliac and Inflamatory Bowel Disease. J Pediatr Gastroenterol Nutr 3:676-682.

46-Schmitz J. 1997. Lack of oats toxicity in celiac disease. Br Med J 314:159-160.

47-Shidrawi RG., Day P., Przemioslo R., Ellis HJ., Nelufer SH., Ciclitira PJ. 1995. In vitro toxicity of gluten peptides in celiac disease assessed by organ culture. Scand J Gastroenterol 30:758-763.

48-Simon O. 1998. The mode of action of NSP hidrolysing enzymes in the gastrointestinal tract. J Anim Feed Sci 7:115-125.

49-Sollid LM. 2002. Coeliac disease: dissecting a complex inflammatory disorder.
Nat Rev Immunol. 2:647-655.

50-Srinivasan U., Leonard N., Jones E. 1996. Absence of toxicity of oats in adult celiac disease. Br Med J 313:1300-1301.

51-Srinivasan U., y col. 1999. Lactase enzyme, detected immunohistochemically, is lost in active disease, but unaffected by oats challenge. Am J Gastroenterology 94:2936-2941.

52-Talal AH., Murria JA., Goeken JA., Sivitz WI. 1997. Celiac disease in an adult population with insulin-dependent diabetes mellitus: use of endomysial antibody testing. Am J Gastroenterol 92:1280-1284.

53-Thaysen EH. 1935. Ten cases of idiopathic steatorrhea. Q J Med 4: 359-365.

54-Thompson T. 1997. Do oats toxicity in celiac disease. Br Med J 314:159.

55-Triboi E., Abad A., Micheleno A., Lloveras J., Pllier JL., Daniel C. 2000. Enviromental effects on the quality of two wheat genotypes quantitative and qualitative variation of storage proteins. European Journal of Agronomy13:47-64.

56-Trier JS., Allan CH., Abrahamson DR., Hagen SJ. 1990. Epithelial basement membrane of mouse jejunum. Evidence for laminin turnover along the entire crypt-villus axis. J Clin Invest 86:87-95.

57-Troncone R., Auricchio S., De Vincenzi M., Donatiello A., Farris E., Silano V..1987. An analysis of cereals that react with serum antibodies in patients with coeliac disease. Pediatr Gastroenterol Nutr 6:346-350.

58-Troncone R., Ferguson A. 1991. Animal model of gluten induced enteropathy in mice. Gut 32:871-875.

59-Van Belzen MJ., Koeleman BP., Crusius JB., Meijer JW., Bardoel AF., Pearson PL., Sandkuijl LA., Houwen RH., Wijmenga C. 2004. Defining the contribution of the HLA region to cis DQ2-positive coeliac disease patients. Genes Immun 5:215-20.

60-Variend S., Placzeck M., Fraafat., Walker-Smith..1984. Small intestinal mucosal fat in childhood enteropathies. J Clin Pathol 37:373-377.

61-Verbeke SP., GotteLand MR., Fernández M., Brunser OT. 2001. Papel del tejido conectivo en la morfología y función de la mucosa intestinal. Su importancia en la patogenia de la enfermedad celíaca. Rev Méd Chile 129:1333-1342.

62-Walker-Smith J., Murch S. 1999. Coeliac Disease. Disease of Small Intestine in Childhood. Fourth Edition. Isis Medical Media Ltd 235-277.

63-Wieser H. 1996. Relation between gliadin structure and celiac toxicity. Acta Pediatr Suppl 412:3-9.

64-Wieser H. 1998. Investigations on the extractability of gluten proteins from wheat bread in comparison with flour. Z Lebensm Unters Forsch 207:128-132.

65-Wieser H. 1998. Investigations on the extractability of gluten proteins from bread whet in comparison with flour. Z Lebensm Unters Forsch 207:128-132.

66-Yu KCW., Mamo JCL. 1996. Killing of arterial smooth muscle cells by chilomicron remmants. Biochem Biophys Res Commun 220:68-71.

www.ingramcontent.com/pod-product-compliance
Lightning Source LLC
Chambersburg PA
CBHW040828180526
45159CB00001B/109